Prayer and Grace

My Journey to a New Heart

Bardolf & Company

PRAYER AND GRACE
My Journey to a New Heart

ISBN 978-1-938842-06-1

Published by Bardolf & Company
    5430 Colewood Pl.
    Sarasota, FL 34232
    941-232-0113
    www.bardolfandcompany.com

Cover design by Michael Cissell

To my loving wife
Cindy
who is always there for me

Jane,

I'm so glad I got to meet you today & I'm glad you have done well during your journey as well. I hope you are encouraged by my journey & writing.

Psalm 20,

Prayer
and
Grace
My Journey to
a New Heart

Steve Burcham

Bardolf & Company
Sarasota, Florida 2013

CONTENTS

ACKNOWLEDGMENTS

I would like to thank:

My friends and family,

My CaringBridge visitors for encouraging me to write,

Cindy for encouraging me to finish the book,

Chris Angermann for transforming my humble writings and shaping them into a story with flow,

All the medical professionals who are now part of my "new family,"

John Ryberg and Asbury United Methodist Church,

Danny Windham and Digium for their extraordinary support throughout my adventure.

FOREWORD

It is my great joy as a pastor to be up close and personal in the high, holy times of the people I love. Some of those moments come disguised as everyday occurrences; some sneak up on us and leave us wondering...what just happened? Others are milestones and ceremonies, placed on the calendar and approached with an array of emotions. In all of these intersections between the divine and the human, I see the faith of my friends not just formed, but revealed.

For years, Steve and Cindy Burcham have lived in the midst of the Asbury church family. They have raised their children, worshipped, served and given generously of their time and talents to grow God's family. Long before they faced the challenges of Steve's failing heart, they distinguished themselves as people with an infectious joy and deep faith. Steve is the kind of guy you ask to lead your finance committee. Bright, generous and organized, he is a rare blend of analytical engineer and faith filled optimist. Cindy is warm, thoughtful, resilient and incredibly strong. And wherever Steve or Cindy engage or commit themselves, you can be sure the other is rock solid right beside them in the trenches.

If they had never been tested by Steve's heart problems, their life would still have been a wonderful testament to God's faithfulness. But in their time of trial, they showed that their faith was not a fair weather love affair with Jesus. Of course, there were low times, when we had every reason to fear that Steve might not survive physically. But even in those times, their faith in the goodness of God was revealed to be well founded.

It seems more than a little surreal to look back on these times. Especially that day, which began with Steve in Huntsville Hospital, included a helicopter ride and ended with him in the UAB hospital heart transplant unit. Some phrases still ring in my ears from that day, "Oh, somebody dropped the ball on the transportation arrangements." "Vital signs incompatible with life." "John, be sure to tell Cindy the important papers are in the desk in the study, in case I don't make it." Throughout that day we prayed, talked and encouraged each other. I admit it; Steve's faith gave me confidence on that difficult day.

But there were very happy times, too. I will never forget the joy everyone experienced as Steve walked his daughter, Lindsey, up the aisle at her wedding. In that moment and so many others, Steve showed me how a person can keep an eternal perspective while living each moment here to the fullest. This is a rare gift and one that I hope to cultivate. These pages reveal Steve's journey, but they also reveal how God sustained Steve and his incredible family through a tough part of that journey. Pay attention, I believe you will find encouragement for your own journey. I did.

The Rev. John Ryberg
Associate Pastor
Asbury United Methodist Church

PRELUDE

STORM WARNINGS

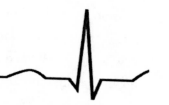

I have been a strong believer in prayer for a long time. That may be an odd admission for an engineer like me, who has been trained in math, scientific formulas and evidence-based truth; but over the years, I have had a number of experiences when I have felt God's presence in times of need. His guidance has not always been easy, but it has never failed me.

Perhaps the most significant occasion pertaining to the events described in this book occurred on January 29, 2008. It happened before dawn in the basement game room of our home in Madison, Alabama. A few years back, I had developed the habit of praying in the middle of the night when I woke up and couldn't go back to sleep. Rather than stewing for hours about things troubling my mind and managing to fall asleep just minutes before the morning alarm, I'd get up and use the opportunity to commune with the Lord.

During the summer when it was warm outside, I'd usually sneak out onto the back deck and enjoy the magnificent panorama of Rainbow Mountain. All of the houses on the west side of Stargate Drive, perched on a small ridge, are blessed with the best view in town. But that winter night the temperature was in the 30s, and I had gone to our basement.

I was praying fervently, in despair about my job prospects and the imminent failure of an important church project. The automotive parts company, where I'd worked for 25 years as the longest running director of operations, had recently been sold. The new owners were looking to reduce costs, perhaps even to shut it down, leaving thousands of employees jobless. At the same time, a much needed, new center for contemporary worship service at Asbury United Methodist Church, whose planning committee I led, was struggling to gain the necessary financial support.

Although I had recognized the signs for both predicaments early on the horizon, I had been unable to do anything productive in the face of the problems growing more acute, and had been praying for guidance about them for months. Now that things were coming to a head, I felt very much at the end of my rope, and was kneeling on the rug, my elbows on the ottoman with my head in my hands. Teary-eyed, I shared how devastated I would feel if I failed as a leader both at work and on an important project of faith.

Suddenly, in the dim glow of the lamp behind me, I felt His presence. It was as if He were right there, kneeling beside me with His arm on my shoulder. I sensed more than heard Him say, "The two things you have been praying about are going to be all right, but there are going to be challenges ahead that sadden me." I felt His sorrow deeply, almost as if we were crying together.

I sprang to my feet, my heart racing, and then quickly sat down in the leather chair behind me. Incredulous, I whispered to myself, "I just heard His voice, He answered my prayer!" I grabbed my Bible, found an old index card inside and jotted down the date and what I had heard word for word. That gave me pause. The Lord said my career and the building project at Asbury were going to be OK, but He was sad about the future. It was an answer to a prayer, but with a caveat. What could that mean?

But rather than dwelling on the negative, I felt excited. I closed my Bible and glanced around the game room, remembering many of the good times my three girls and their friends had had there, playing pool and foosball, watching movies and hanging out. One year, they painted a winter wonderland mural on the south wall, and it had been hard for my wife, Cindy, and me to paint over it during a recent remodeling. Dismissing the strange caveat for now, I smiled and thought, "Many more good times to be had down here."

As I headed upstairs to get dressed for work, I felt invigorated and hopeful again about my future. Little did I know that He had something else in mind altogether, something that would strike me to the core of my physical and spiritual being.

CHAPTER 1

BEGINNINGS

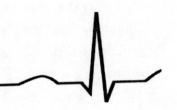

I grew up in the southeastern section of Huntsville, Alabama in the late 1960s and early 1970s. My dad was a civil engineer by training and worked for the space division of the Chrysler Corporation. It is a little known fact that one of America's big three automakers had several companies, one of which built the early Saturn rockets. My dad was the first in a family of farmers to go to college, and he believed in the importance of education. He stretched the family budget to buy a house in the Grissom High School District, an upscale part of town, so that my brother, three sisters and I could benefit from its institution of secondary learning. Grissom High School was named after Virgil "Gus" Grissom, the astronaut who perished in the Apollo 1 fire at Cape Kennedy in 1967, and was considered one of the best schools in the state.

But while all of us received a good education, there was not much left for other conveniences. As a teenager, I shared a bedroom with my brother. Our split-level suburban home had one telephone on the kitchen wall for us kids to share. It did have a long beige receiver cord, though, so my sisters could speak to their boyfriends while sitting on the steps leading down into the den, where no one else could listen in. At a time when most of my schoolmates had color televisions in their homes, we made do with a 13-inch, black-and-white model. We were "house rich" and amenities poor.

My mom, Marjorie, who had been Elizabeth Taylor beautiful when she married my dad, was prone to depression. As many women diagnosed with "mental problems" during that era, she received electroshock treatments and often sat around the house medicated, in a world of her own. I remember spending nights and weekends visiting her when she was hospitalized during one of her many crises and wishing she could be healthy and active like the moms of my friends. Being robust and energetic myself, I vowed that I would never be a burden on my family.

When it came to spending money on extras like a new bicycle or go-cart or motorcycle, the cash had to come from the fruits of my own labor. From the time I was old enough to throw our local newspaper, *The Huntsville News*, onto people's front porches from a bicycle, I had a job, sometimes two or more at once. I knew early on that the only way I could succeed in life—get what I wanted—was to work and study hard, and I was proud to be independent and self-reliant from an early age.

When I turned 16, I asked one of the ladies on my paper route about a car that sat idle in her driveway—a 1967 Plymouth Barracuda Notchback, Army green on the outside, black vinyl on the inside. I had had my eyes on it for some time. She and I agreed on a payment plan, and for $225—one dollar per cubic inch of engine volume—plus the cost of a few accessories from JC Whitney and a new coat of paint, I discovered a newfound mobility and freedom.

Cruising around town with my friend Duffey one day, we noticed a construction trailer in the parking lot of a strip mall. When curiosity got the better of us and we inquired what was going to be built there, the man inside, Mr. Dampier, hired us on the spot to do construction clean up. By the time I was a senior, a jewelry catalog showroom opened up there, and I received my first promotion—from sweeping the floor to selling diamond rings, bracelets and necklaces behind the glass countertops. It meant donning a suit and tie, and I felt duly self-important.

There were other kids from my high school working part-time at the store, too. One of them, a cute brunette at the service desk, caught my eye. Her name was Cindy. There were just 15 feet of carpet-covered concrete between the two bullpen showcases and countertops where we worked—15 feet of space traversed by a split-second glance and smile sent her way, with Cindy occasionally reciprocating.

Sometimes our department manager, Mr. Boffa, leaning on one counter or the other, would be caught in the middle and notice our teenage exchanges with a smile of his own. Another salesman, Kevin, saw the developing magic, too—as well as the problem: My timid nature around a pretty young woman was causing me to miss out on an opportunity.

One night, Kevin nudged me into action. Grinning from ear to ear, he said, "If you don't go ask her out on a date right now, I will," and started moving toward her desk. After a moment of panic—and the accompanying adrenaline rush—I bolted in front of him and broke the ice with Cindy!

For our first date on January 19, 1980, I took her to Shoney's Big Boy, and right from the start, she never let me forget how cheap I was. Afterward, we went to "1941," a comedy starring

John Belushi, and we had a good enough time that when I dropped her off on her parents' doorstep later that evening, she agreed to another date the following weekend.

Somehow we survived those unimpressive beginnings and became high school sweethearts. Not long after, Mr. Boffa and his wife invited us to their house for dinner in order to encourage our budding relationship. Although introverted in public, Cindy opened up quickly once she got to know someone, becoming bubbly and outgoing. She had a positive, can-do attitude like me, and would tolerate no nonsense. Because of her pretty, round features, she was known as "chubby cheeks" among her close friends. She was a good sport about the nickname, but woe to anyone who couldn't resist pinching her cheeks in endearment: It would earn him a quick punch to the gut that knocked the breath out of him—as happened to my neighbor, Steve Breland, and me on separate occasions. (Fortunately, we were both quick learners and never experienced Cindy's fisticuffs prowess again.)

When it came time for college, Cindy and I both went to the University of Alabama in Huntsville. Following in my father's footsteps, I studied to become an engineer and eventually got a master's degree from Auburn University. When we got married on June 1, 1985, Cindy quit school so we could start a family, and we were soon blessed to have three wonderful daughters, Lindsey, Brooke and Anna.

I knew that I would have the role of primary breadwinner. I wanted my daughters to have a solid foundation for success—a college education—so we started to save and invest to make sure we would have the funds necessary to make that happen. But there was considerable division of labor in our family: Cindy managed the household, which included the finances; so I made the money, and she told us how to spend it.

I started working for Chrysler as a junior engineer during my sophomore year in college and continued with the company after graduation. Moving up in the ranks, I ended up running the manufacturing plant, Automotive Electronics City in Huntsville, where I was in charge of more than 2,500 employees in two buildings, including a large segment of unionized workers. We shipped over 30,000 electronic units per day—to more than a dozen automobile factories in North America.

To be closer to my workplace, we moved to Madison, a small town west of Huntsville. It was founded in the early 1800s and was then known as Madison Station, a train depot servicing the surrounding farming community. When we arrived there, it was still a quiet, agricultural town—I affectionately refer to it as "Mayberry"—but the westward rush of young professionals soon swelled the population tenfold, and today it is a bustling community with national chain restaurants, supermarkets and superstores like Lowe's and Walmart. Still, Madison hasn't lost its small town charm. The mayor and members of the city council show up at homecoming football games, and are happy to invite you for breakfast or lunch if you wish to chat with them about the town and its future.

Perhaps the most significant change in my life, my spiritual development, occurred after we settled in Madison, first on Siena Vista Drive and later in a house we built on Stargate Drive—and I credit Cindy for it most of all. When I was growing up, we were not a particularly religious family. It would have been unusual if my parents took us to church more than five times a year. Sunday was just another day of the week. What little foundation I had up to this point was the result of the efforts of others, not my family or the church. I remember when I was in fifth grade, the after-school 4-H club leader helped me "let Jesus into my heart." In seventh grade, a friend, Jesse May, taught me how to pray during a sleepover one night. And when I was in 10th grade, Mrs. Fleming, who owned a large estate on Whitesburg Drive, challenged me in front of her family and friends when I stopped by to collect my newspaper fee, asking, "Son, do you believe in our Lord Jesus?"

When Lindsey was little, at Cindy's prompting, we started to look for a church that would reflect our values. We visited a new upstart church on Hughes Road and later learned that the founding pastor, Marcus Long, lived around the corner from us on Siena Vista Drive. In the afternoons, he began to stop by in his green Volkswagen Bug to pay us visits. After a few conversations, we felt that we had found what we were looking for and decided to join Asbury United Methodist Church. It was 1988, and I still remember Cindy, with Lindsey in her arms, and me being welcomed at the front door by Richard, a greeter, while Bill, an usher, frantically scrambled to find us a place to sit in the already full fellowship hall, which was serving as the temporary worship area.

Marrying Cindy and getting involved with the staff and congregation at Asbury were the keys to maturing me. In many ways, we all grew up together. We built our own home, and Asbury expanded and moved into its own place of worship. The Asbury family helped raise our three beautiful daughters.

From 2000 to 2010, at the prodding of Ted, our youth leader, Cindy and I volunteered in Asbury's youth department, Fathom Ministries. Looking back, this was the best decade of serving ever, bar none. Starting with Lindsey's seventh-grade age group through Anna's 11th-grade year, we did whatever was required. We oversaw the department's finances, delivered food, ushered Wednesday night Fathom meetings, taught Sunday morning school, led Sunday night small groups, drove the vans, went on domestic and international mission trips and retreats, and actually intervened in a few troubled-teen episodes.

I found out quickly that the kids were not shy to pray for each other either in public or private—they simply "got it." They became models for me, although it took a while before I was confident enough to follow their example, to "kick it up a notch" and take my approach to prayer to the next level.

Although I was on a path of spiritual evolution, it wasn't until several years later that I experienced the real power of prayer and made it a habit to communicate daily with God in order to seek His guidance. In time, I also came to realize and believe that He speaks to us and answers our prayers in many ways—through scripture, movies, books, people and sermons; and directly during prayer, in gentle nudges, slight almost inaudible whispers, and for me, also through dreams.

It took even longer for me to understand that self-sufficiency and self-reliance will only get you so far in this life.

During the time I was climbing the corporate ladder, Cindy was busy both as a homemaker and a community volunteer. She worked in the nursery and Child Development Center at Asbury, taught preschool, carpooled the kids to The Dance Company in Madison, volunteered at their schools from kindergarten to grade 12, and shuttled them and their friends to band, softball and cheerleading events. Cindy helped me teach youth Sunday school, something I wasn't initially comfortable doing. She baked and delivered food for Sunday morning Sunday school and Sunday night small groups, and was always "there" for the girls and their friends when they needed her. Along the way, every night, we shared a hot home-cooked meal as a family.

While I worked to be the breadwinner, she managed to put twice as many miles on her car every year than I did on mine. She endured my out-of-left-field excursion for a season or two as a part-time Amway salesman on top of my demanding job. And, in the mid-90s, when my career looked like it was going to take a detour through Detroit, she happily supported the idea to the point that we went house shopping north of Motown for a weekend. A timely job opening at the plant kept me in Madison.

In 1998, Daimler-Benz, the German conglomerate best known for making Mercedes cars, acquired Chrysler. It was a big international story, but for us at Automotive Electronics City, the impact was negligible. Nothing changed in the way we did business until 2004 when we were sold to Siemens, another German mega-company that supposedly had a better understanding of automotive parts manufacturing and the electronics industry. I was the only senior staff member who stayed on and became a key player in ensuring a smooth transition. But our success was short-lived. In 2007, Siemens sold the company to Continental Automotive. Managing a unionized labor force in times of uncertainty and cutbacks proved demanding—by then we were down to 1,700 employees—but I have never walked away from a challenge, and I thought things were going reasonably well. So I was surprised when at the beginning of January of the following year, I was offered an early-out severance package. It was generous and befitting my years of service to the company.

When I discussed the offer with Cindy, she was dead set against it, arguing that I had too much invested in the plant and that we owed much of our life to my working there. I explained that this change in ownership was more serious than the previous time and that such a lucrative package would not be available later on. Knowing me well, Cindy figured—correctly—that I had made up my mind already, and although she acquiesced, she did so under protest.

The following Monday, I popped my head into the office of the VP in charge and told him I would accept the early-out package. But my assuredness that we would be able to step out on faith without a firm landing pad was not nearly as strong as I had given Cindy to understand; which is why I ended up praying in my basement later that month for spiritual help and guidance.

My confidence in the Lord was rewarded and true to His promise, things worked out well quickly. When I put out feelers to my friends in the area's aerospace, defense and telecom industries, it took less than three weeks to get a positive response. On Valentine's Day, I got a call from the CEO of Digium, Inc., an up-and-coming company in the unified communications industry. He offered me a job as director of quality and we quickly settled on terms. I said good-bye to a quarter century career in the automotive world at the end of April. I was surprised by the large going away party the company threw for me, which included many of my current and past colleagues and mentors. Two weeks later, on May 12, I started my new job at Digium.

I soon realized how lucky I was to get out when I did. Within several months of my departure, the bloodletting began.

A number of my former colleagues departed and found jobs in defense and aerospace. Others were terminated and moved away. Some of them were fortunate like me and ended up at Digium.

In less than two and half years, the new corporate owner shut down Automotive Electronics City for good, gutting the plant and moving its product lines to other plants in Texas and Mexico and ridding management of the burden of having to deal with a unionized labor force.

Whenever I had occasion to drive past the shuttered gates and concrete barriers that blocked the entrances to the parking lots, I felt sad. Another American manufacturing icon fallen to the relentless corporate quest for double-digit profits. When I worked there, the plant and talent were second to none. I know this firsthand because in my senior position, I had the opportunity to tour similar facilities in Mexico, Canada, Germany, the United Kingdom, the Czech Republic, France and Malta. It was never about a lack of technology or know-how. The reason for the shutdown was to pursue cheaper manufacturing opportunities in other regions of the world. Although that chapter of my life is closed, it left me with an unpleasant aftertaste.

In the meantime, the other major challenge in my life was helming the expansion of Asbury Church. I had sat on a previous planning committee to raise funds and oversee a new prayer center, only to see the project fail miserably. The estimated costs were simply too high. In addition, plans called for building in what turned out to be the wrong location, across the street from the new youth center and the large parcel of land the church had recently acquired. To no one's surprise, after considerable wrangling, the project was dead in the water.

I should have known better when plans resurfaced a year later, but I allowed myself to be recruited to lead the committee. Although I vowed not to find myself in the same predicament as my predecessor, I promptly got pulled into a vortex of similar squabbles. By the time everyone had added the things to the building they wanted, it had grown into another unfeasible mega-project with an astronomical, unrealistic price tag. I felt that my leadership was on the line. I didn't want to be the second guy in charge to fail.

After my nighttime encounter with the Lord, however, I had a newfound confidence. I decided to get angry and flex my leadership muscles, insisting that we scale back the project to what our pastor needed right then and there—a new worship center and enough space for Sunday school with the children. Meeting with the architect, I made the necessary changes unilaterally, pushed hard for approval and got it done. It didn't hurt that my new boss at Digium contributed a handsome sum to the building fund and that another parishioner and his daughter gave $1 million after I took them to lunch, laid out the plans and explained what we needed. That contribution moved us past the goal we had set to allow us to start construction.

So far, everything the Lord had told me had come to pass, but what about the caveat? Several events transpired that I interpreted as possible reasons for His expression of sadness.

In July, we had a terrible scare with our daughter Lindsey. She had always had a small freckle on her chest, but when she returned from her first year of college, it had grown bigger and discolored. At Cindy's insistence, we took her to a specialist, Dr. Gray, for a biopsy. When we went back for the results, the doctor and nurse came into the examining room pale-faced and delivered the news that it was melanoma. They talked to us as if Lindsey were a dead person walking. Needless to say, my daughter was as frightened as they were.

I took a deep breath and insisted that the doctor and nurse give us some time alone. Then I knelt in prayer with Lindsey and asked the Lord for help and guidance. Miraculously, He reappeared. Once again, I felt His presence close by, assuring me that this was not a big deal. I heard Him say distinctly, "Pray and minister to them. Have courage, show your faith."

And that is what I did, both for Lindsey and the medical practitioners. Dr. Gray not only removed the melanoma and a large area surrounding it successfully, but also did a terrific job as a plastic surgeon, so that the incisions remained virtually invisible to the naked eye. Although that crisis ended happily, it gave us enough of a scare to make me wonder if it weren't perhaps what had saddened the Lord when He'd come to me.

Another possibility concerned our family assets. While I insisted on fiscal responsibility on the Asbury project, I didn't take my own advice when it came to my own finances. I had invested my entire 401(k) rollover in the stock market, only to see it all disappear during the economic downturn when General Motors went belly-up. I was devastated when it happened, and it has taken us some time to dig out of that financial hole.

Also that fall, Cindy's grandfather died at age 97. Gramps, as we called him, had lived in Daytona Beach and had a great sense of humor. I still remember him back in the early 90s sending me a birthday card with four scantily clad women riding Jet Skis on the ocean. He had covered the photo with typed notes to me, in effect concealing them in case Cindy was looking over my shoulder when I opened the envelope. The note read that the picture was part of a study he was conducting to see how much fabric was required to hold swimsuits in place, and that he had already learned that not much was needed, but the study must continue "for scientific reasons." Even though Gramps had lived a full life, he spent his final two years mostly asleep in bed in a nursing home. It was a sad occasion for all of us, and we continue to miss him and Gram dearly.

Still, as we were heading toward Christmas, our lives were back on even keel. Yes, we had experienced some sad times, but things were definitely looking up. By then, I was well integrated into the corporate culture of Digium, with weekend slow-pitch softball games and other employee outings. Being part of a growing company that appreciated its employees was exciting. I was also looking forward to breaking ground on the new campus at Asbury after the New Year. It felt good to be once again a successful business executive and a respected leader at my church. Our children were doing well in school, and my wife was a great mom and cherished community volunteer. We were living the American Dream—hard work and good values paying dividends—with a sense of fulfillment in all of our endeavors.

Then, late in December, I woke up one night and after tossing and turning for a while, decided to get up and pray. This time, I headed to my study in the front of the house.

When we built our home, the architect designated the room just to the left of the entrance door as the parlor. To me that meant, "formal room that will never be used." So I lobbied for it to be my study. I insisted on masculine décor—dark, textured, painted walls with heavy crown molding, a built-in wooden bookcase and my mahogany desk in the center. Usually, I'd just grab one of the chairs in front of the desk, turn it toward the window and the amber glow from the street lamp outside, and sit and pray in the semi-darkness before going back to bed.

On this particular night, the second I sat down, I felt nervous and uneasy. As I started to pray, I felt even more unsettled and my heart started to race. Suddenly, I felt the Lord's powerful presence. This time there were no words of advice, just a message in the form of an indistinct vision, something foreshadowing a coming health problem, an organ failure of some kind.

I don't remember how that session ended, only that I felt troubled, but not afraid. I knew, as I returned to the bedroom, that I would not be able to get back to sleep.

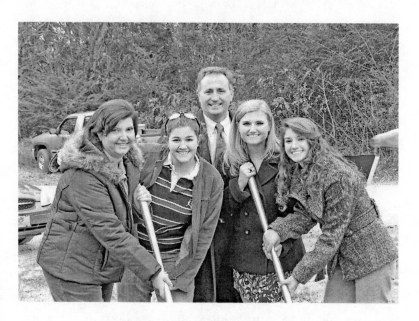

From left: Cindy, Brooke, me, Lindsey and Anna
at the ground-breaking for Asbury's new campus

Chapter 2
First Signs

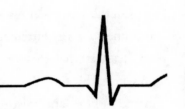

In January of 2009, I was climbing up and down a stepladder to trim the crepe myrtle in our front yard when I felt a tingling in my arms. It was an unpleasant, prickly sensation as if my limbs had fallen asleep. But it went away and didn't recur, so I dismissed it and didn't think anymore about it.

The first indication that there was something seriously wrong with me occurred a month later. I had taken some accrued vacation time to accompany Cindy and our youngest daughter, Anna, on a three-day weekend to the National Cheerleading Competition, which was being held at the Wide World of Sports Resort in Orlando, Florida.

My oldest daughter, Lindsey, had made a point that I never seemed to make time for her regional band competitions, and Anna had chimed in about how I hadn't made a national cheerleading event so far, so I acted like I let her twist my arm and came along. Secretly, I enjoyed it a great deal.

Anna was a flyer for the Bob Jones Patriots' Competition Cheer Squad—one of the people who gets lifted and tossed in the air. I remember when she was four years old, carrying her around the house holding her stiffly upright by her ankles. By the time she was 11, she would scale the arched entryway in the kitchen like Spider-Man, all the way to the top of the nine-foot ceiling. She'd surprise us perched there—I never figured out how she did it!

We arrived Friday afternoon and settled in for the weekend competition when some of the best squads in the nation would go up against one another. Parents and chaperones at these events essentially serve two purposes: 1) Make sure the girls are where they are supposed to be, on time, in the right cheer uniform and mood; and 2) get to the arena early dressed in school garb, save seats for all the parents and cheer like crazy when the girls hit the mat. Saving seats was a little too confrontational for me—the competition among cheer parents can be fiercer than the contests on stage—so I usually found other things to do, like "parking the car," while the stands were being flipped between performances.

Anyone who thinks cheerleading is not a sport needs to spend only a little time with the girls to change his mind. They work tirelessly all year long on routines that last all of two and a half minutes—concentrated athletic feats that require strong, flexible bodies, stamina and artistic flare, not to mention nerves of steel. So we were proud parents when after two days of flawless performances consisting of squad tucks, full-ups, handsprings, basket tosses and more, the Bob Jones squad was rewarded with the winners' "white jackets." (For Anna, who was a sophomore at the time, it was the second in what became a collection of white championship jackets.)

The awards ceremony on the mat in the middle of the arena was utter pandemonium, with coaches beaming and a horde of parents snapping photos. Afterward, the winning and placing teams milled around talking to each other and swapping team souvenir shirts. When the chaos finally settled, we all headed to the Ale House for some burgers, fries and a late night celebration.

Monday morning I rolled out of bed before sunrise to pack up the rental car and drive to the airport for an early return trip. We wanted to be ready when Anna arrived with the team on a later flight to attend a celebratory victory reception at the Huntsville airport that evening.

Getting the suitcases downstairs and into the trunk proved to be more of an undertaking than expected. Returning to the room, I told Cindy, "I feel weird. My heart is racing and I just got winded pulling our two suitcases to the car."

"Well, we only had four hours of sleep last night. Maybe your blood sugar is low," she said. "Let's get to the airport. You can get some juice and fruit. Maybe that will help."

Reassured, I went back to the parking lot to pull the car around while Cindy finished checking out. It was still dark outside, and I felt a little disoriented as I drove to the front of our hotel in the Wide World of Sports.

As I sat there waiting, my cell phone rang. It was Cindy. "Steve, where are you? I'm standing out front waiting for you!" her voice crackled.

"Well, I'm right here staring at the front door. I can see the brightly lit front desk and you are nowhere to be seen. Are you sure you are standing out front?"

"*Am I* sure I'm standing out front? *Are you* sure you're waiting out front?" she replied more tersely. "Steve, where are you? I'm really standing here all alone."

I replied, "I'm waiting, engine running, right in front of..." and I read the sign: Wide World of *Music*—oops!

"Sorry, I'll be right there to get you, honey," I said sheepishly.

When I made it to the right place and Cindy got in the car, she asked, "Are you sure you're OK to drive?"

"Yes," I answered as we departed the Disney complex and headed for Orlando International Airport. "I just turned right instead of left, and all these buildings look the same, you know."

The flight back was uneventful, and we made it home without a hitch. We had lunch, unpacked and retrieved our wiener dog, Dixie, who was happy to see us despite being spoiled by grandparents in our absence. Then we headed back to Huntsville International Airport for the arrival of Anna and her victorious cheerleading squad. But as we turned into the the entrance and divided highway leading to the airport buildings, suddenly, without warning, my heart started to race.

I said to Cindy, "There's that weird feeling again," and then everything went black.

I remember her crying out, "Pull over!" and then nothing.

It couldn't have been more than a few seconds that I was out because as I regained consciousness, I heard Cindy shout, "I've got the wheel! Please take your foot off the accelerator."

When my head slumped sideways against the headrest, she had grabbed the steering wheel and guided the SUV for me.

I managed to pull over to the breakdown lane and put on our flashers.

"What happened?"

"You passed out! We are going to the emergency room right now. There is something wrong with you."

I didn't want to miss out on Anna's homecoming celebration, but my feeble protests that I was OK really fell on deaf ears. Cindy insisted on switching places with me and drove to the hospital in Huntsville.

Before long, I was sitting in an emergency triage room, hooked up to monitoring equipment.

Soon, Anna arrived at the hospital, too, having missed out on the festivities at the airport. As soon as her plane had landed and she turned on her cell phone, she got Cindy's message about my "heart attack." At Cindy's request, our friend Buddy was waiting for her in the arrival lounge. The happy homecoming quickly transformed into puzzled looks followed by prayer huddles on the part of the team and coaches as Buddy whisked Anna out of the terminal and on to see me.

By then my symptoms had abated, and all my vital signs, based on an electrocardiogram (EKG) I had received, were fine. I was already looking forward to going home when the attending cardiologist arrived looking concerned.

When I told him I felt fine now, he said, "Mr. Burcham, being winded, disoriented and blacking out is serious business. I would like to keep you overnight for observation. We'll get an echocardiogram and perform a heart catheterization tomorrow to check for blockages and overall heart function. Does that sound OK to you?"

What could I say, except yes, although I lodged a minor protest, saying, "I've never had high cholesterol or anything like that."

Watching my heart beating on the viewing screen during the echocardiogram later that night reminded me of the sonograms we had done during Cindy's pregnancies, although it was an odd sensation seeing something inside myself "out there." I became fascinated by the chambers and valves all busy pumping in synchronized harmony, moving oxygenated blood to my body and brain and spent blood to the lungs for resupply. I felt His presence that night as I marveled at His creation and felt as excited as a kid examining a caterpillar under a magnifying glass for the first time.

The next morning, as I was being wheeled on a gurney into the catheter lab, I felt a bit on edge. Somehow it had all begun to sink in. I was 46 years old and had never had an occasion to visit a hospital except when Cindy gave birth to our three daughters, and to visit a sick friend or family member. The idea that I was ill, perhaps seriously, didn't sit well with me at all.

The nurse spread a sterile, blue paper blanket over me, and I was fully awake as the doctor inserted a port into an artery in my groin just above the right thigh and guided the catheter all the way to my heart. When he went about measuring pressures and looking for blockages, I suddenly started to feel queasy.

"Doctor, there it is again, that feeling!" I exclaimed.

He stopped and looking at the monitor screens, said, "Oh, that's a classic atrial fibrillation pattern. You've got AF. We can treat that. Everything else looks fine; all pressures are within normal range."

I didn't know whether to feel good or bad about that news, but his matter-or-fact attitude reassured me.

That afternoon, I checked out with a prescription for calcium channel blockers and a follow-up appointment scheduled for a month later to discuss the possibility of having a cardiac ablation procedure to fix the AF. It would be done just like the catheterization, except that the doctor would look for "electrical shorts" in the heart and then use radio frequency radiation or alcohol to disable the offending area of the heart muscle, removing any shorts in the tissue permanently, thereby correcting the AF.

I felt more confident by then and was a bit irritated that I was not allowed to walk out on my own, having to endure being wheeled to the discharge area by a volunteer despite my insistence that I was fine. "Safety rules and insurance matters," I was told.

"Hospitals!" I thought with a sigh, not realizing then how well I would get to know them down the road.

CHAPTER 3
COMFORTABLY IN DENIAL

The doctor at the hospital had warned me that the medications might have some side effects, and they did. I felt tired and winded at times, as I complained to Dr. Drenning, the senior cardiologist at The Heart Center whenever I went for a checkup, but I didn't let those symptoms slow me down at work, and there was no recurrence of the lightheadedness that had brought me to the hospital in the first place.

So in early March, when our friends Buddy and Carole invited us to go with them on a ski trip to Utah, where they own a timeshare, I checked with Dr. Drenning to make sure it would be OK. He was a serious athlete himself, going for 15-mile bicycle spins on the weekends. In his late 40s now, he had competed in the XTERRA World Championship and actually won the Ironman competition in Hawaii. Lean, chiseled and sinewy, he could be a bit brusque, but after examining me thoroughly, he cleared me for the trip.

Although Cindy decided to stay home to catch up on work, I was looking forward to spending time with Buddy and Carole and our daughter Brooke. It was my first snow skiing trip out West, and I had never seen treeless snow-capped mountains before.

Buddy, Carole, Cindy and I actually went to the same schools together, but we were only acquaintances. When we moved to Madison, they happened to live in the same neighborhood, and we just clicked. We started going on vacations together when the kids were still babies and continued to do so when they were grown. They're both athletic—they were competition swimmers and hooked up as lifeguards at a neighborhood pool—and are always fun to be around. We would do anything for one another.

We arrived at the condo in Utah late Saturday night, and I took over the kitchen on Sunday morning. On weekends at home, I always cook up a hot breakfast, and continued the tradition, waking the late sleepers with the overpowering smells of bacon, eggs, pancakes, grits and coffee. After everyone was well fed, we all suited up and hit the slopes.

It was a picture-perfect day—the early sun was bright, the sky a knockout blue—as we unloaded at the top of the ski lift. We had dropped off Brooke in a half-day adult ski class. The rest of us sporty types took to the more serious slopes. Buddy is the most proficient skier among us, followed by Carole and me. I like green, blue and double blue runs, and an occasional black diamond if it's fairly free of moguls.

We decided on a combination of three runs for our warm-up, and started to traverse the slope to the top of the first. I immediately got winded, so much so that I had to stop to catch my breath. I didn't think I was that badly out of shape and blamed the medications on my inability to exert myself.

Carole was aware of my condition and stayed behind with me when I stopped repeatedly going down the runs. At one point, she skied up to within a few feet of me and stopped, dusting my boots with snow. She leaned on her poles and said in a concerned voice, "Steve, are you sure you are OK? I can't remember you ever struggling so much. We can go back to the lodge and rest a while—I can catch up with Buddy later and ski until lunchtime."

I wasn't ready to throw in the towel. "No, let's both catch up with him. I can make it. I just have to take it easy."

So we continued and had fun. Even with periodic rests, the morning flew by in no time.

At lunch, we joined the horde of other skiers at the lodge in line for food and drink. The midday sun was hot and we enjoyed our meal at one of the outdoor, slope-side tables.

After we finished, I took our trays to the receptacle by the outer wall of the lodge. By the time I got there, I had to lean on the trash can because I was so winded. Back at the table, I took my pulse. It was 55 beats per minute, much lower than usual. I searched "heart rate" on my smartphone and scanned a few articles from various cardiac centers; I discovered that the normal range for a human heart at rest is 60 to 100 beats per minute. I was below that, a condition the articles called "bradycardia," in which not enough oxygen gets pumped to the heart, resulting in faintness and shortness of breath; but it's not serious unless the heart rate dips below 50.

Not a problem. I figured the thinner air at our high altitude was to blame and decided to soldier on. So we geared up for an afternoon on the slopes and had a fine time, with me taking it easy.

Returning home, I considered the weekend a great success and figured the heart ablation would take care of things.

But three weeks later, while sitting at my desk at Digium, I started to feel faint. I waited for it to pass, but it didn't. When I measured my pulse, it was 44 beats per minute.

I put in a call to The Heart Center and got my usual nurse, Tiffany. She asked me to come to the center right away to run some tests. She and I had a good, kidding relationship, although she wouldn't put up with any "feeling sorry for yourself" attitude, which suited me fine—most of the time. While I was hooked up to the EKG machine, she and I caught up on my skiing trip and the latest antics of her son, Cooper, a two-year-old little dynamo at the time.

While she took the printout to show to the doctors, I checked my e-mails and texted Cindy to bring her up to speed on what was happening. She was away with Anna, attending a leadership conference at the University of Alabama in Tuscaloosa.

Suddenly, the door flew open and Tiffany entered with a nurse practitioner in tow. They both had serious expressions on their faces.

"Steve, you are in full atrioventricular heart block," Tiffany informed me. "You need to have a pacemaker installed. The doctors will be in to see you momentarily."

"A pacemaker. You're kidding me, aren't you?" I exclaimed.

When tears started to well up in my eyes, Tiffany quickly said, not unkindly, "Man up, Steve. Pacemakers are no big deal. We have babies with pacemakers!"

I took a deep breath. "OK, OK, but can y'all just excuse me for a minute while I get my head around the news?"

"Sure, but make it fast. The doctors will be here soon."

As soon as I was alone, I prayed to the good Lord for His wisdom, healing power and guidance. I called Cindy and Buddy. Even though Tuscaloosa was under take-cover severe weather warnings, Cindy decided to leave the conference early and return to Huntsville to be with me.

Soon, Dr. Drenning arrived with Dr. Allison, an electro-physiologist, who gave me the rundown on what was happening to me. Apparently, the AV node, the electrical connection between the atrial and ventricular sides of my heart, had quit working. The heart is like a dual pump, with the atria keeping the ventricles primed, and the latter doing all the work. In my case, with the AV node being blocked, the ventricles didn't know when to beat, so they were operating at a default rate, called the "escape rate."

"It's sort of God's backup system keeping you alive at forty-five beats per minute," Dr. Allison explained.

Everyone's escape rate is different, and some people walk around with it for years without showing any symptoms. But I led an active life, so that wouldn't do for me. I would need a basic pacemaker to reconnect the two sides so they could operate normally again. The procedure was simple—nothing extreme like open heart surgery—and I would be in the hospital all of two days, mostly for observation purposes. An operating room had already been scheduled for me the next morning.

Once I gave my consent, they left, and I just sat there staring at the floor, with my head in my hands.

"Steve, are you OK?" Tiffany's voice sounded concerned.

I looked up and managed a grin. "I guess so. I just need to get used to the idea, right? I mean, who wants to have hardware installed in their chest?

By the time Cindy got home from Tuscaloosa, I had made my peace with it. We didn't talk about it other than to confirm that it was a routine procedure and the thing to do. I can't say I slept very well, though, and I spent a good deal of the night in my study praying.

My support network went into action, though. The next day, shortly after I was admitted to the hospital, Buddy called and we discussed if I would still be able to scuba dive after the implantation. We were both "Open Water II" sport divers, which meant we were certified to 130-foot depth, and he knew this was important. He did some quick research and determined that, barring other health issues, it would be possible depending on the type of pacemaker. One manufacturer's device was good only to 60 feet of depth, but another worked down to 300 feet.

When I told my nurse, he wrote a gigantic message on my chart that the surgical team couldn't miss even if they had blinders on, and they installed a pacemaker "compatible with my lifestyle."

I sent the nurse a thank you note, and later he was recognized as "employee of the month." Aiding me with my request probably wasn't the first time he went above and beyond the call of duty to help a patient under his care.

As promised, installing the pacemaker went off without a hitch. Dr. Allison performed the procedure. In his early 40s and the antithesis of Dr. Drenning—smiling, personable, with a good sense of humor—Dr. Allison had been an electrical engineer at Alabama Power like me before he went to med school, which may be why we got along so well.

Being knocked out, I don't remember any of the installation of the pacemaker, of course. There was little discomfort afterward, and the results were great. For the first time in three months, I didn't get winded at the slightest exertion or feel faint. As an engineer, I was not just personally but also professionally impressed by the amazing technology available, which previous generations couldn't even imagine.

I was delighted to be able to get back to all of my old routines with family and friends. I sent Dr. Allison a card to thank him for curing me and turning me into a bionic man by installing this electronic device in my chest—better than new.

The only warning came in the form of advice given during my inaugural morning run as I resumed my three-times-a-week workouts with my running partners, Dee and my neighbor Steve (also known as "Tire Boy" because he owns a handful of area automobile tire stores).

We made our way down to the lake in our neighborhood, stopping periodically to stretch both our legs and arms in preparation for the run. During our final break, I was in my own little world, staring at the ducks paddling on the water with ever-expanding ripples in their wake. Tufts of fog were rising from the surface of the water, and with the sun still hidden behind Rainbow Mountain, the faint light promised another low-humidity, crystal clear, blue-sky day ahead; and I thought, "I couldn't have asked for a better morning for my inaugural run with the guys!"

I had missed our sessions and it felt good to get back in the groove. When it was the three of us, I let Dee, who is a few years our senior and a good foot taller than me, and Steve, who is my age but already sports a full head of salt and pepper hair, run up front together while I quietly brought up the rear. They usually talked incessantly about books they'd traded, dissecting the storylines as if they were the greatest plays by William Shakespeare. I waited until they tired of that before changing the subject to current events.

That first day back, I felt so frisky that I decided to change the routine a bit by running circles around them—literally—

while they were engaged in conversation. I'd pass them on the left, then cross in front before dropping back on the right behind them and repeating.

It took only three loops before Dee looked over and asked, "Steve, did you ever figure out why youre AV node failed and it required a pacemaker to fix it?"

As we slowed to jogging pace, I replied, "No I did not. According to the doctors, an AV block is not uncommon, so they installed this electronic bridge with batteries good for eight years. Who really cares why I needed it? I'm fixed now."

"Well, I think you need to go to the University of Alabama in Birmingham for evaluation to see if they can figure out why all this happened," Dee insisted.

Tire Boy added, "Yeah, I see Dr. Bourge there for dilated cardiomyopathy. He says I may need to start working on my diet and take some medication to head off any future issues. They really are experts there."

"Thanks, guys, I'll consider it," I said, "but I'm feeling absolutely back to normal now. I'm not sure if knowing the clinical reason why I had to have this gadget implanted would change anything for me. It's doing its job just fine, 24-7."

They nodded and we returned to our normal pace.

In retrospect, I should have listened to them, but at the time I was flying high, basking in the return of my health and energy. I figured that the sad, ominous messages I received during the special prayer sessions when I felt the presence of the Lord were all about going through this episode, and that was the end of it.

And for a number of months, it was.

CHAPTER 4

FIRST BRUSH WITH MORTALITY

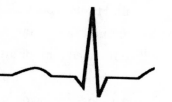

In August, I went on a wonderful scuba diving outing with Buddy to Key Largo in Florida. We did eight dives over the course of two days without the slightest problem. We saw stoplight parrotfish, trumpet fish, grouper, and four-eyes, and followed a six-foot green moray eel for some time. We swam through three long caverns in the reefs, and on a deep drift dive in a strong current, managed to photograph three spiny lobsters and some spotted scorpion fish.

The fall passed uneventfully with football games at Auburn. College game days in the South are a lot of fun. When the Auburn Tigers played at home, Cindy and I would drive there on Friday, enjoy the company of our daughters and return to Madison late Sunday. By mid-December, with eight wins on the scoreboard, Auburn was slated to play Northwestern in the Outback Bowl on New Year's day.

Around that time, I got my annual allergy-induced sinus infection. The usual over-the-counter remedies didn't work—I kept feeling lethargic and was running a fever. We were planning to spend Christmas vacation in St. Augustine, Florida with Cindy's parents and siblings, and I didn't want to suffer throughout the holidays, so I went to see my primary care doctor in the middle of the month.

Dr. Graham was around 65 years old and had just about seen it all. He also spent his personal time helping the needy in our community and in impoverished countries throughout the world. I appreciated him for his punctuality and no-nonsense approach. He'd typically do a little bloodwork, make an assessment, give you a shot of some drugs and send you on your way. In this case, he wrote me a prescription for two five-day packs of azithromycin to take back to back and told me to come see him again if they didn't do the trick.

The following afternoon I went for my first "device check" at The Heart Center. It had been six months since Dr. Allison had installed the pacemaker. When I got there, I noticed Cooper, Tiffany's young son, running down the hall. It turned out that Santa had come for a special holiday visit, and staff members brought in their youngsters after school to see him and receive presents.

Soon I was sitting back in as comfortable a chair as the center provided—not very—hooked up to a computer that allowed a technician to take the "vital signs" of my pacemaker.

"Everything looks fine, Mr. Burcham," he said, looking over the printout. "Overall performance is good, and there are no recorded cardio events in the device's memory. We'll see you again in six months."

My early present from Santa!

I was really looking forward to spending time with Cindy's folks, although the drive to St. Augustine seemed interminable.

Cindy's mom, Eve, and stepfather, Dr. Owen Garriott, the hosts for this family get-together, had rented a big two-story house on stilts right on the beach. It has an ocean-side deck complete with walkway and steps bridging the dunes down to the sand just yards short of the Atlantic. Dr. Garriott is a retired astronaut who had spent time aboard the Skylab space station during the 1970s.

It was going to be a house full of kids, from Cindy's young nieces, Arden and Marin, to her sister's children, Bryan and Allison, both pre-teens, to our three teenagers. Cindy's brother, Billy, is a mountain bike enthusiast. You wouldn't think he would have much opportunity to pursue his passion in Florida—not exactly known for its mountain terrain—but it turns out there are some great courses in abandoned coquina quarries with black diamond challenges. I was also looking forward to finding out what kind of specialty beer he had put in storage. Not a fan of "lite beer," Billy goes for dark and exotic brew.

We took our suitcases to our bedroom upstairs and settled into catching up with all of the family.

Unfortunately, even after eight days of antibiotics, I didn't feel any better, although I managed to enjoy the mayhem of the opening of the presents on Christmas morning. With the sunlight reflecting off the Atlantic and brightening the great room, I sat back and soaked in the sounds of paper tearing, boxes being pried open and the occasionally muttered "Aw, thank you, I love it," punctuating the general chaos. The kids were really digging into the piles of presents under the tree.

Dr. Garriott gave me a signed copy of his book, a hardcover he'd published about his adventures aboard the Skylab. He and his fellow astronauts were making history running and performing experiments on the newly orbiting space station, although it was somewhat crippled at the outset. One of the solar panels and a heat shield hadn't opened during the initial deployment, creating all sorts of challenges for the crews to sustain their activities.

Toward the end of the present-opening frenzy, Bryan asked if we could set up his new BB gun target range downstairs, and I immediately agreed to help. It had been a long time since I had shot a BB gun, and it was as much fun for me as for him. After I had my fill of target practice on the sandy ground underneath the house, I decided to head back upstairs.

Much to my chagrin, it was a struggle to make it up to the deck. My limbs felt like rubber, and I had to stop every few steps to catch my breath.

Cindy appeared on the deck and asked me what was wrong.

"I can't make it up there," I told her. My second Z-Pak of antibiotics ran out today."

She met me, put her arm under one of mine and helped me up the steps.

"What do you think I should do?"

"Find a doc-in-the-box first thing in the morning."

As I sat waiting at the emergency care clinic in St. Augustine the next day, I was hoping that perhaps another course of more powerful antibiotics would finally knock out what was ailing me.

The doctor entered with my chest X-ray in his hand and put it up on the viewing screen. We spent the next few minutes marveling at the see-through image of my pacemaker. The microchips, capacitors, battery and resistors inside were all clearly visible, and the wires running through the heart valves connecting to the tissue walls reminded me of telephone wires strung between poles.

Everything looked normal, but then the doctor pointed out, "Your heart is large. Look how big it is in the chest cavity."

"Yeah, everyone says I have a big heart," I quipped with a grin.

The upshot was that he gave me a prescription for a five-day course of ciprofloxacin and told me to come back to see him if that didn't do the trick.

I thought to myself, "Hmm, heard that one before. Let's hope these meds work better."

But they didn't. I spent the next few days mostly sleeping and holed up in our upstairs bedroom reading a tattered copy of "Moby Dick," the only "manly" book I could find in the bookcase. Once in a while, I'd get up for a bite to eat.

After taking the last dose of the antibiotics, Cindy and I decided to cut our family visit short and return to Madison. By now it was clear that there was something seriously wrong with me, and if a hospital stay was in my future, I'd rather be home than in a strange place. I managed to reach the nurse in Dr. Graham's office on the telephone and scheduled a visit first thing the next day.

Dr. Graham came into the examining room, greeted me and started poking and prodding my torso. Then he put his stethoscope to my chest to listen to my heart. As usual, he got real close, his head no more than five inches from mine. As he listened, his neutral expression turned into a frown and his bushy eyebrows furrowed.

He jerked back all of a sudden, pulled the stethoscope out of his ears and said quite loudly, "How long have you had that *thing* installed in your chest again?"

"Oh, a little over seven months now," I replied, "Why?"

"You've got a heart infection, probably endocarditis. I can hear the inner wall of the heart rubbing against the outer wall with every beat!"

While he left the room to call Dr. Allison at The Heart Center, I searched "endocarditis" on my smartphone and managed to pull up some ugly looking images. Uh-oh. This seemed like something that would be very difficult to treat. "Scraping fungus from inside the heart," didn't sound like a walk in the park. But it did explain why the antibiotics had been ineffective.

When Dr. Graham returned, he said, "Steve, I just got off the phone with your cardiologist. He wants to see you right away."

At The Heart Center, an EKG revealed acute pericarditis with me being close to tamponade—the condition in which pressure builds up because of fluid in the space between the heart muscle and the pericardium, the outer sac covering the heart. When the pressure outside becomes greater than inside, it renders the heart's pumping action ineffective and, without intervention, is fatal.

As he explained the situation to Cindy and me, Dr. Allison said, "Your general practitioner is quite perceptive having found this; but it's not endocarditis, a very difficult condition to treat."

In fact, Dr. Graham had saved my life. Our respect for our family doctor went up several notches.

"Pericarditis is easier to treat," Dr. Allison continued, "but you'll have to be admitted to the hospital right away for an emergency pericardiocentesis."

Dr. Allison had already scheduled an operating room for that evening. "You'll wake up with a thin tube protruding from your chest allowing the fluid to drain," he explained, adding, "You'll need to be here for several days to allow for follow-up care."

Then he turned to Cindy and said, "Due to the serious nature of this condition and considering the holiday, I am admitting him directly to the Intensive Care Unit, which means limited visitation, but round-the-clock monitoring.

There was little time to process any of this. I could tell Cindy was shaken and teary-eyed from the barrage of information being thrown at us.

"While you're here, I'm going to call in an infectious disease doctor to see if we can find out why this happened, OK?"

I nodded, and thought to myself, it was a good thing he hadn't added, "Happy New Year."

I was knocked out for the procedure and came to only long enough to then drift back to sleep; but when I woke up on New Year's Day, I felt like a burden had been lifted from me. For the first time in weeks, I was myself again.

By the afternoon I was sitting up in bed, energized and ready to conquer the world. Auburn was playing Northwestern in the Outback Bowl, and I enjoyed the game in good company. Asbury's associate pastor and a good friend, Brother John, Cindy and Anna had come by the hospital to keep me company. So did the nurses and technicians who were loyal Auburn fans like me. They kept "visiting" my room—I was the only lucid patient in the intensive care unit that day—to watch the game in progress.

It was close to half time when Dr. Allison appeared. Smiling broadly at the assembled crowd of spectators, he said, "How do you feel after having one full liter of fluid drained off your heart, Steve?"

"Much, much better."

He came over to my bed and, brandishing a giant syringe, said, "If your football friends want to hang around, that's OK with me, but I need to get what final bit of fluid I can off your heart and pull this tube out."

Judging by everyone's interest in the game, not to mention their curiosity about the tube and valves protruding from just under my sternum, no one was going to leave the room during the procedure. It was a bit like fans looking forward to watching the commercials during the Super Bowl.

When Dr. Allison first connected the syringe to the tubing and pulled the plunger back, no fluid came out. He then pulled the main tube out of my chest about an inch—surprisingly, it didn't hurt at all—switched several valves and pulled the plunger out again. This time some fluid emptied into the catch container. He repeated the process several more times, with everyone watching intently. One time, he forgot to switch the valves in the correct sequence, and when he went to empty the syringe into the catch basin, bloody fluid shot across the room in a mighty spurt onto an adjacent countertop.

"Oops," he said, as the spectators laughed nervously.

Shortly thereafter, he declared he was done and pulled the tube all the way out of my chest. It was 10 inches long, with tiny perforations along the final five inches, like a miniature garden soaker hose.

"I'll send this fluid to the lab for analysis. You can stay here another hour or so and finish watching the game, but then, with the nurses' help, get up and walk around," he said.

He promised to stop by later to see how I was doing. If I felt good, I'd be moved to a regular room. "An infectious disease doctor will take over from here," he continued. "He'll likely want to take additional blood samples for culturing, so plan on being here a few more days."

"Thank you for the warning, Dr. Allison, you've worked your magic again," I said as he left uttering, "War Eagle," the Auburn Tigers' battle cry.

A "few more" turned into five days. During that time, I was "worked up" by the infectious disease doctor, and tested for everything from AIDS to leprosy. Some of the detailed questions bordered on the ridiculous, and severely tried my patience. Cindy and Brother John were in the room when I gave the doctor an exasperated look and said, "I'm a white, monogamous male. I've been married to or dating the same girl for 31 years. I don't sleep around or shoot up drugs, so get on to the next category, please."

The story must have made its rounds through the hospital, because Dr. Allison mentioned it, chuckling, when he went over the test results with me. All of the indicators had come back negative.

"I guess your bout with pericarditis remains a mystery for now."

"Par for the course," I replied, "'Why' seems like an unanswerable question for me lately."

With that I got my discharge papers and marching orders. I was scheduled to see him and Dr. Drenning in a month to find out how things were progressing.

"This could have been an acute episode, or you may have developed chronic pericarditis. If that's the case, we may have to go in surgically and make a small window in the bottom of your pericardium to allow fluid to drain continuously," Dr. Allison told me. "But we'll cross that bridge if we have to. Please don't worry about it now."

Chapter 5

Slow Downhill Run

If I hadn't had my daily prayers to keep me on a steady course, I don't know what I would have done during the roller coaster ride I was on for the next year and a half. For a while, I'd feel perfectly fine; then I'd have a period when I experienced shortness of breath and fatigue. Return visits to my cardiologist would result in a new diagnosis with associated medicine and diet changes. Then things would return to normal again, only to plunge into another relapse. I kept the Lord apprised of my worries, hopes and wishes at night and during my early morning prayers. Although He didn't make Himself known to me as before, I still felt a powerful connection that made it possible for me to get through the day at work and on weekends, even during times of flagging energy and frustrating setbacks.

There were some good times and happy milestones along the way. Asbury's new Grace Worship Center had its inaugural service on Easter Sunday, April 4, 2010. The week before, we had held a small commissioning service with a few key church members and supporters who helped make it all happen, and I was gratified that all the hard work had finally come to fruition. In the name of the Lord, and with His help, we had created something we all could be proud of.

My three daughters were all doing well. By late spring, Brooke returned from her sophomore year at Auburn. Anna applied for and was accepted into an internship at HudsonAlpha Institute for Biotechnology, which kept her busy during the summer. And newly graduated, Lindsey had landed her first job at Quorum Business Solutions in Houston, Texas. Cindy, Anna and I helped Lindsey move into her first apartment close to work in a nice section of town called the "Galleria Area." I had mixed feelings the day we returned home to Alabama without her, just as I'd had after dropping her off for her first day at Auburn—happy that she was a successful young professional, and sad that she was moving so far away to get her career started.

But my health was another matter.

I went on a jog with Carl, the manager of Digium's technical customer contact center in San Diego, California. I had been promoted to Vice President of Operations and Quality recently and picked up responsibility for his group along the way. I had not managed customer contact centers before, and now I was actively overseeing two of them. Carl was a young, technically capable manager. He was in town for a week of leadership team building and training. When he let on that he liked to jog, I invited him for an after-work run on the Indian Creek Greenway Trail. The two-mile, paved sidewalk winds alongside the stream that roughly defines the boundary between Huntsville and Madison and is a popular place for people who stroll, walk, bike and rollerblade, while enjoying a pleasant view of a wooded, hilly area to the east and farmland filled with grazing cattle to the west.

As we stretched and warmed up, I uttered a "pre-game" warning: "Carl, this old guy here has had some heart problems and has a pacemaker. I'm going to give this the old college try, but we may need to back off if I run out of steam."

We took it easy and made it to the turn with ease. But just a bit after the one-mile point, I became winded and motioned to Carl for us to slow down. We reduced our speed to a fast walk so I could catch my breath. I noted wryly that last year around this time, I could still run two miles without stopping, pacemaker and all. Since my bout with pericarditis, my stamina was at an all-time low.

Walking allowed Carl and me to talk, and I learned he was a budding believer. I think he may have been a bit surprised that his new boss was someone who didn't mind talking openly about his own faith. On our way back to our cars, I decided that while our outing had been less than stellar in the jogging department, it was a success after all. We had had a good bonding experience, and it marked the beginning of a friendship that soon extended beyond a merely collegial working relationship, with Carl and me texting one another across the country—I rooted for him in his new, often overwhelming responsibilities as support center manager while he encouraged me to be strong in the face of my health challenges. Even though the passages and messages varied, the themes were the same: stay focused on our Lord Jesus, and we'll both get through all right.

As the summer and fall went by, I found it increasingly difficult to maintain my physical regimen. Not being able to keep up with my friends on outside runs, I spent more time at the gym. I could still jog on the treadmill, but whenever my heart rate approached 150 beats per minute, I'd start to get winded. Even late in the year, I still managed to jog for upward of half an hour at a 13-minute-mile pace, although I would feel lightheaded and dizzy for some time afterward.

I often woke up with shortness of breath in the middle of the night. Getting up helped, but lack of sleep exacerbated my feelings of chronic fatigue and tiredness during the day.

My doctors were now saying I had a little hypertrophy of the left ventricle. This was a condition in which the heart muscle stiffened, preventing the chamber from filling fully with blood between beats. This caused mitral valve leakage and a drop in pumping efficiency, called "ejection fraction of the heart," which invariably led to symptoms like chronic fatigue, shortness of breath, reduced exertion tolerance, dizziness and lightheadedness.

The treatment consisted of a daily regimen of an ACE inhibitor, a beta blocker and a diuretic. I loathed all three pills because they caused my blood pressure to plummet and made me tired and lethargic—hardly an improvement over my heart condition. The diagnosis had changed—from supraventricular tachycardia (SVT) to atrial fibrillation (AT) to bradycardia to pericarditis. Being an engineer with an interest in facts, I read up on those and other heart conditions on the Internet and discussed what I found with my doctors, but while I knew these terms meant something specific to my physicians regarding treatment, to me they were just medical gobbledygook—fancy sounding labels that didn't bring any relief.

I often felt like an old man before my time.

My new role in the company placed more demands on me. I accompanied Digium's management team on a week-long trip to London for a conference with our international distributors. I was fine for the duration, and we all returned home excited, with many ideas to increase our sales and market share in the region. Another trip to China went well, too.

But in late December of 2010, while waiting for an interviewee to arrive at Digium, I suddenly experienced extreme dizziness, tunnel vision and numbness in my right arm and hand. I managed to find a substitute to conduct the interview and went to the ER. An EKG, echocardiogram, chest X-ray and various labs showed mild left ventricle enlargement and hypertrophy. But the physician who took care of me recommended no treatment other than continued monitoring by my electrophysiologist and cardiologist, which I was doing already.

And so the roller coaster of heart issues continued.

During my February visit to The Heart Center, I complained to Dr. Drenning of tingling in my hands and feet, which seemed to be more pronounced at night. On the two or three nights a week when I'd wake up short of breath and fatigued, it would get worse throughout the day. I felt winded even doing light chores like taking out the trash, washing the car or mowing the lawn. One time at the gym, I almost fainted on the treadmill as my heart rate shot up to 180.

Looking tight-lipped and concerned as always, Dr. Drenning suggested that I might be suffering from amyloidosis, an incurable condition in which proteins build up abnormally in the heart muscle, causing harm.

Frustrated, I took to the Internet to find answers. For my next visit toward the end of March, I came armed with printouts of materials I had gathered from various websites and presented Dr. Drenning with *my* diagnosis.

"All things considered, it seems as though I have a developing case of hypertrophic cardiomyopathy (HCM), not amyloidosis as you suggest. I have five of the six symptoms for HCM and only two of 13 listed for amyloidosis."

Dr. Drenning pursed his lips and nodded. "Steve, I know you have HCM. I'm trying to figure out why. If Dr. Allison and I continue to treat you here, our next step is to rule out amyloidosis. But frankly, I think it's time for me to refer you to another center more equipped to deal with this. Your condition seems to be a bit out of our wheelhouse here in Huntsville. I would suggest trying the University of Alabama at Birmingham."

Wow! Dr. Drenning, one of the senior cardiac doctors in the area throwing in the towel. That wasn't very comforting. There was a moment when I felt panicky and downright abandoned, but then my survival instincts took over and I regained my usual composure.

"OK, I agree and I appreciate your offer. But please refer me to the Cleveland Clinic in Ohio. During my research, I've learned that they're experts in treating HCM."

Dr. Drenning looked relieved. "Done," he said.

As he left the room, he added, "Since you like to surf the Web, go ahead and pick the doctor you would like to be referred to, and I'll take care of the rest."

I thanked him and started to get dressed. As I buttoned and tucked in my shirt, I thought, "Maybe now we'll get to the bottom of this."

If you google TripAdvisor for Cleveland, you'll find 70 great things to do there, from theaters, museums, ballparks and the zoo to the Rock and Roll Hall of Fame. But during my first visit to the Ohio city on Lake Erie, Cindy and I skipped the sightseeing attractions. After the drive up from Madison, we checked into the Renaissance Hotel, close by the Cleveland Clinic, and had a nice dinner at the Italian restaurant adjacent to the hotel lobby.

The next morning, we walked to my appointment with Dr. Klein. Entering the premises of the clinic, I was reminded of a modern airport complete with concourses, restaurants and shops, the only difference being that waiting rooms, offices and labs replaced the gates and planes.

Dr. Klein was a senior cardiologist who had published books on HCM and associated treatments. I had actually given Dr. Drenning another doctor's name, because in my wildest dreams, I didn't think I would get an appointment with someone so high up on the totem pole. So, when someone from the clinic called and said my requested doctor wasn't available and that Dr. Klein was going to be seeing me, I was elated.

He immediately put us at ease when he said, "Mr. Burcham, I have reviewed your referral file. You've driven a long way. What would you like to accomplish on this visit?"

I told him at length about what had happened to me over the past year and where I had left things with Dr. Drenning at The Heart Center. He listened without interruption and then typed into his computer while outlining a course of investigation and treatment. He ordered an X-ray, blood labs, echocardiogram, CT scan, and stress and lung tests, culminating in a heart catheterization and biopsy the following afternoon, which would include taking five tissue samples to determine if I had amyloidosis. He also recommended having genetic testing done during my stay to see if I had any one of the 18 gene mutations known to cause HCM.

"Within two weeks, I'll be able to send you a full report outlining my assessment and a treatment plan going forward," Dr. Klein said confidently.

"Sounds great, let's get going," Cindy and I said simultaneously.

He handed me a stack of printouts for my appointments and labs and we departed the examining room heading for our next "gate."

For the rest of the day and the next, I submitted to the battery of tests, after which Cindy and I drove back home, hoping for the best.

Two weeks later, as promised, Dr. Klein called with the results. The good news was that I did not have amyloidosis, and the genetic tests were inconclusive. But as far as what was causing my condition, he was as much at a loss as his predecessors. He said that my heart disease had not "fully presented itself," and told me to come back and see him nine months later at the beginning of the following year. For all practical purposes, I was back to square one with no more answers than before.

And the roller coaster ride continued.

In June, I managed to play 18 holes of golf with my daughter Brooke. Although she beat me with her overall score, I was proud that I outplayed her on the last two holes. I took my final shot, 80 yards away from the green. It made a perfect arc, hit the pin, shaking the flag, and dropped straight down into the hole—an eagle. It was the first time I had ever hit the ball directly in the hole without a bounce on the green— unbelievable! Needless to say, I hopped around grinning from ear to ear like a kid who had just hit the winning home run in a Little League baseball game.

We spent the Fourth of July with Buddy and Carole and the kids on our annual water ski outing at Lake Guntersville. When it was my turn, Buddy kicked the V6 engine of his red and white Sea Ray into gear, and I popped out of the water easily. Concentrating on the slalom run ahead, I passed through the narrow twin markers at the entrance of the course and immediately swung out far right to pass by the first outermost buoy. Then I cut across the boat's wake and, dropping my shoulder closer to the water's surface, successfully passed the second buoy on the other side.

But by this time, I was having trouble breathing from the exertion to the point that I was huffing and puffing hard. As I approached the next buoy, I realized I'd taken too much time recovering and pulled hard on the rope to make up some of the distance and stay on course. Fat chance. I completely lost control and skipped, rolled, tumbled over the water, eventually coming to rest face down. My head throbbed and I had a few body aches, but I was still in one piece. I rolled over and, hyperventilating from the run, just floated and stared up at the crystal blue summer sky.

It wasn't long before Buddy pulled up beside me. "Are you OK?" he asked concerned.

When I grunted, "Yes," he said, while grinning from beneath his light blue Destin Fishing Rodeo cap, "That run was a five but the wipeout was a ten!"

With his help, I pulled myself aboard, still panting heavily. "I think I'm OK...but I'm really...short of breath...a lot more than usual," I gasped, musing that most of the time it was my arms and legs that gave out, but today my entire body had betrayed me.

In early August, we took our daughter Anna to Auburn for the beginning of her college years. We parked the SUV and a

U-Haul trailer filled with furnishings on the sidewalk that ran between the new brick dormitory buildings on the campus and started to unload.

I would have liked to help carry in the bigger items, but Cindy and Anna took the easy chair and relegated me to bringing up a comforter in a plastic zipper bag that weighed only a couple of pounds and other lightweight objects. Even so, after a couple of trips I was badly winded and happy when Cindy declared that a trip to the TigerTown shopping center was in order to pick up some necessary items. I welcomed the air conditioning and the opportunity to take it easy later that afternoon at Brooke's place while Cindy and Anna finished getting Anna's dorm room into shape.

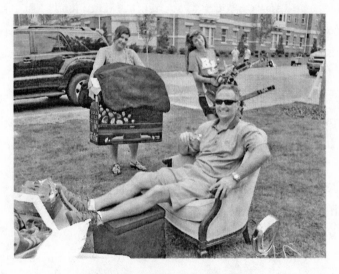

Clowning around, but unable to help
moving Anna in at Auburn

And that was me on a good day—because by that point in late summer, I was fatigued most of the time. I felt sluggish and "full," as if I had just eaten a large meal. I no longer slept in my bed because I would wake up feeling like I was drowning. I'd spend the night upright in my easy chair in the den, sometimes leaning forward on a pillow in my lap just to be able to breathe.

I could no longer scuba dive, run or jog, much less carry heavy loads or push a loaded wheelbarrow up an incline. Managing to walk to the car or climb a flight of stairs without stopping became an impossible chore. One project a day was my limit before exhaustion set in.

The rales in my chest got worse, and I had to leave work several afternoons to go home and take a nap. Sometimes, I'd break into uncontrollable fits of coughing. Once it was so bad that I gave myself a hernia, which was an even more painful condition than my heart disease. Twice I ended up in the emergency room at Huntsville Hospital for intravenous diuretic treatments to remove fluids that had built up around my organs. I felt better both times, but only for about a week or so.

I kept thinking that if my HCM wasn't that bad and there was nothing else wrong with me, why couldn't I run, jog or do physical labor as I was able to do even a year ago?

When I went to see Dr. Allison at the beginning of September, I inundated him with a litany of complaints, concluding, "Since the Fourth, when I couldn't even complete a slalom water ski run, I've been sliding downhill health-wise and the slope is getting steeper every day."

"Steve, I've reviewed the last quarter's worth of test data on you," he replied. "It looks like you have a full blown case of congestive heart failure heading toward end stage."

I shook my head in disbelief. "Congestive heart failure? End stage? Isn't that what happens to older people after they have been fighting heart disease for decades? How can I go from having some "simple electrical problems" a few years ago to CHF today? The Cleveland Clinic said it would be years before my disease fully manifested itself. It's only been four months since that visit!"

"There's always a next step, Steve," Dr. Allison said gently.

He went on to explain that in my current condition, I needed a new pacemaker, a device with a built-in defibrillator that could shock the heart back into rhythm when it stopped or tried to "tach out." Apparently, most people with HCM had a pacemaker implanted as a safety precaution. He recommended one that would provide "bi-ventricular pacing," which would re-synchronizing the chambers of the heart and improving pumping efficiency.

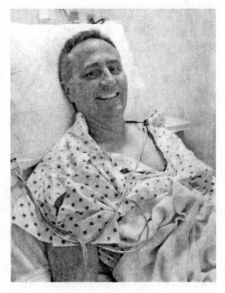

I was familiar with end-stage treatment of CHF from papers I had read on the Internet and knew he was right, so I agreed to have the replacement done. I resigned myself to living with the hernia a bit longer, since I would have to wait six to eight weeks after the procedure to get it surgically fixed. Dr. Allison promised no miracles—no surprise there—but insisted

In the hospital, after I got my new pacemaker

that often these devices made a huge difference in improving quality of life.

Two months later, at the end of October, we went for a weekend visit to Auburn for a football game. Brooke had plenty of room at the condo, so we stayed there with her.

We came up early on Friday, and I helped her with yard and house maintenance work while Cindy spruced up the interior and reloaded the refrigerator. We took Anna, Brooke and some of their friends to the Mellow Mushroom that evening for pizza and beer.

On game day, we loaded up on Daylight Donuts for breakfast, packed the coolers and found a good parking spot at the stadium. We visited other tailgaters, connected with old friends, and watched the Tiger Walk, a special pre-game event in which the band, team, cheerleaders and coaches parade down Donahue Avenue into Jordan-Hare Stadium.

An hour before the game, we started the trek up the hill and up the ramps to our seats on the 50-yard line in the upper deck.

Before we left for the weekend, I had written Dr. Allison another thank you note. I wanted him to know that the new pacemaker was making a huge difference in mitigating my symptoms. To test it further, I decided to climb to the upper deck of the stadium without stopping.

As I ascended the ramp and enjoyed the Auburn campus coming into fuller view below in the afternoon sun, I felt no shortness of breath. I turned back to Cindy and said, "Hurry up! The heart patient is beating you to the top!"

She didn't change her pace, though, and continued to talk to the Morrises, the parents of Anna's boyfriend, Jake, who had joined us for the day. By this time, Cindy knew all too well that I had both highs and lows, so she knew better than to celebrate an apparent improvement when there invariably would be another setback around the corner.

Not me, though. As an incurable optimist, I relished the return of my vitality.

"I made it!" I exclaimed as we reached our level. Among the chaos of fans crisscrossing every which way on the concourse to grab a soda, popcorn or pretzels from the concessions stands, my spontaneous outburst went unnoticed.

The group caught up and we headed over to the breezeway leading to our seats. At the other end of the short tunnel the opening grew wider, and the brilliant green field came into view. Players were warming up, stretching and tossing footballs, getting ready for the kickoff.

I'm feeling good again—finally!" I thought.

Chapter 6
Second Brush
with Mortality

It turned out that Cindy was right, as usual. A week after the Auburn game, when I was almost convinced that the pacemaker was a miracle cure, I began to experience congestive heart failure symptoms again.

Cindy and I travelled to Texas to help Lindsey move from one apartment to another in preparation of her fiancé, Jay, joining her there after their wedding in December. Between the pain of my hernia and my renewed shortness of breath, I was unable to carry even a bag of groceries inside from the car, much less move any furniture items. So we didn't object when Lindsey contracted movers to do the heavy lifting, reducing our job to bringing in knickknacks and organizing everything in her new place.

I was sitting on the couch, recuperating, when Lindsey rushed in white as a sheet and spluttered, "Mom had an accident, I'm about to faint!" She sprawled on the floor while I ran outside. Cindy was in the apartment breezeway covered with blood, a large clay planter in pieces at her feet. Carrying it from the SUV, she had tripped on a raised section of sidewalk and fallen. The planter had burst into many sharp shards on impact, which had given her puncture wounds in her chest, left wrist and right underarm. Lindsey turned away when I helped Cindy through the door and started first aid. Fortunately, things looked worse than they were. Although she was in considerable pain, none of the wounds needed stitching up.

Cindy was healing well but still a bit sore on the Wednesday in November when I went into the hospital to have my hernia taken care of. I opted to have a spinal block anesthetic rather than being intubated and put under completely. In my experience, it made the recovery period a lot easier because the body didn't have to get rid of all the powerful knockout drugs. The operation went without mishap and when the surgeon examined me in the early afternoon, he declared the hernia repair a success and released me from his care. I was looking forward to going home, but the nurses in the post-op area told me I wasn't going anywhere until I urinated, demonstrating that my kidneys and bladder were working again after the spinal block.

By the time six-o'clock rolled around—closing time in the postoperative area—I still hadn't managed a successful trip to the bathroom, and the nurses had no alternative but to admit me for observation. Later that evening, my kidneys and bladder obliged and functioned just fine, but I had to resign myself to waiting until Thursday morning to be released.

Considering it was the hospital, I had a comfortable night, but when I woke up, I felt short of breath. The nurses called in Dr. Drenning for consultation. After a quick examination, he concluded that the intravenous fluids I had been given during the surgery were now overloading my heart and prescribed a few rounds of diuretics to help drain them off. That meant I would probably be able to go home the following day.

Sure enough, on Friday morning I woke up feeling great. I got out of bed, took a shower, shaved, got dressed and nibbled at the institutional lunch while waiting for Dr. Drenning to stop by to give me the quick once-over and clear me to go home.

Cindy, who had been keeping me company, was reading her Kindle when Pastor John arrived. He had heard my short visit to the hospital was turning into an extended stay and wanted to look in on me on his way to prepare for a wedding rehearsal that would take place at the church later that night.

John was a former Marine and still sported a crew cut. He was about a foot taller and wider at the shoulders than me and might have been considered intimidating if he didn't always have a smile on his face and a twinkle in his eyes. Before he had decided to go into the ministry, he and his petite wife Beth owned and operated a restaurant. Now they both worked at the church and occasionally recruited me to help with small maintenance tasks around their home, a service I was happy to provide in return for a cold beer afterward!

We talked about Lindsey and Jay's upcoming wedding, which John would officiate as well, and how much I was looking forward to seeing our oldest daughter getting married.

"But don't let me keep you," I concluded. "We should be out of here shortly, just waiting on the doctor now."

The second those words left my mouth I started to feel dizzy. I pushed the lunch tray away, drew my legs up on the bed and leaned back. "Whew, that's weird. The bed is spinning like I'm drunk. I feel like I'm going to pass out."

Cindy sprang into action. "I'll grab the nurse," she said and headed for the door.

She soon returned with Dr. Drenning in tow. As soon as she saw me, she pointed at the side of my neck and exclaimed, "Doctor, take a look at his neck. His veins are bulging! You can see his heartbeat right there!"

Dr. Drenning said, "Steve, you are distended, overloaded with fluid. Your heart is working too hard right now. Get out of those clothes and back into a gown. We'll take you to the catheterization lab. I need to measure your heart pressures and output before you go anywhere."

Within minutes two nurses came into the room to prepare me for an emergency catheterization. As they began to shave the right side of my groin area above the thigh, where the port would be inserted, I said, "I've been peeing all day; I'm concerned about needing to go to the bathroom during the procedure."

"It's only thirty minutes, Mr. Burcham," one of them said. "Are you sure you can't make it that long? Otherwise, we'll have to insert a Foley catheter 'you know where' and hang a bag."

"I know the option," I replied. "I've just got a strong feeling this is going to take much longer than thirty minutes today."

After they finished inserting the catheter, Cindy and John returned to the room. While we waited for a lab to become available, I was treated to a succession of my friends making their way to my bedside. Somehow they had learned of my deteriorating condition and had come over to try to comfort me with jokes, encouragement and prayers. Nothing worked, however. I was in a very weird state, freezing cold one moment, burning hot the next; faint and dizzy; lucid and wired. I felt like I was on one of those carnival rides with little round modules spinning on a large, rotating platter that tilts at ever more precarious angles; only my ride had the additional joy of sometimes passing under intense heat lamps, sometimes under arctic air conditioning vents. Brother John and Cindy were busy daubing my forehead with a cool washcloth and fetching me tiny cups of water to sip while I struggled with the symptoms of cardiac shock.

It was freezing cold later on, too, when I finally lay on the operating room table for the heart catheterization, squinting at the bright lights above while trying to pick up clues from Dr. Drenning, hunched over to my right and collecting data via the catheter in my thigh. Based on my first catheterization, I was expecting some feedback in the way of readings and assessments, but he said nothing, just concentrated in silence. Then he looked up at me with the most concerned look I have *ever* seen on his face.

"Steve, these readings are not good," he said. "Your heart is shot, done. You need a new one, a heart transplant. I'm calling the University of Alabama in Birmingham and transferring you there tonight. I'm leaving the port in your leg for continuous pressure monitoring and to administer intravenous medications. Right now, we'll get you up to the intensive care unit for stabilization until the transfer is approved and transportation services comes to get you."

"Heart transplant! Did I hear that right?! I was ready to *go home* this morning, and now he says I need a transplant? There's no way I'm getting a transplant," I thought.

But then a new sensation took over. As the nurses wheeled me out of the lab, I couldn't feel my arms and hands from the elbows down. It was like they'd been amputated.

Later that evening, still freezing cold, with my hands and arms numb, I was lying in bed in the intensive care unit. Brother John was holding my left hand and we were reminiscing about our friendship and our favorite scripture. By this time, I was getting a little confused. I could remember the gist of my favorite verses, but was completely off the mark with the references. I attributed verses from Ephesians to Luke, and John gently corrected me. His presence was keeping me together physically and spiritually.

At some point Anna rushed into the room. Carole had intercepted her as she was returning home from Auburn for Thanksgiving and had brought her to the hospital. Arriving in the ICU waiting room, she had stopped dead in her tracks, shocked at the number of family and friends with forlorn faces already gathered there. Before she had a chance to speak to anyone, Brother John, who had momentarily left my side, greeted her in the guest lobby to bring her to my room to see me. On the way, he did his level best to comfort her and prepare her for what she was about to see, but Anna wasn't buying it. Entering the room, she joined my dad, his wife, Sara, my brother, his sons, and Cindy, who were gathered by my bedside. Like them, her face scrunched up as she greeted me and tried to hold back her tears.

"I must really look terrible if they're all reacting to a visit with me like that," I thought.

Eventually, the nurse caught on that John was violating the "two visitors at a time" rule and shooed everyone but him and Cindy out.

At the time I didn't realize that they were saying their farewells, and that was probably a good thing. Eventually, it occurred to me that John was missing his wedding rehearsal to stay with me, and I am forever glad and grateful that he did.

One of the nurses entered abruptly and declared, "I just checked with transportation services. Someone at shift change dropped the ball. The ground ambulance has now been changed to air. A helicopter and medical team will be here shortly for you, Mr. Burcham."

When the flight crew arrived, dressed in their helmets, suits and special gear, I thought we were going into outer space. Yet, their can-do competence was reassuring somehow, although the pilot indicated that with the night's headwinds, it was going to be a bumpy 45-minute trip instead of the usual 30-minute flight. When he asked whether I were prone to motion sickness and wanted to be sedated, I told him that I was a scuba diver and deep-sea sport fisherman and had never gotten sick, even in the roughest of seas.

"Great," he said. "Team, load him up, and let's go!"

Moments later they had me shoehorned into the left side of the chopper with the pilot on the right and two flight-qualified nurses behind me. Space was so tight I figured if anything happened to me during the trip, all they'd be able to do was watch and pray. We quickly climbed into the moonless, star-filled night sky, and I dozed off as the Huntsville lights faded from view. The next thing I remember, seemingly just moments later, was the faint glow of the sodium-vapor city lights of Birmingham. They became larger and brighter until I could make out streets and buildings, and finally the landing pad on top of the hospital complex.

As the rotors sputtered to a standstill, I could see a guest service employee pushing a gurney toward the aircraft. The scene was brightly illuminated under the helipad floodlights. I was actually a bit more aware again, although I felt like I was lying on a bed of ice. It didn't help when the cold air rushed in under my blankets as I was being unloaded.

The pilot climbed down and walked around to the passenger side, shook my hand and wished me well. Noticing his graying hair and weather-worn skin, I thought that he probably had earned his stripes and piloting skills flying sorties in Vietnam.

Once I was secured on the gurney, I was whisked inside and ferried down long corridors. At some point, there were gigantic golden letters on the wall: HEART TRANSPLANT INTENSIVE CARE UNIT.

"Those words again, 'Heart Transplant,'" I thought. "Not me, not now!"

As I was being guided through the door of a hospital room, I saw a team of nurses and residents gathered around a tall man in a white coat. He had a full beard, a balding head and an olive complexion and reminded me a bit of Sammy Sosa, the baseball player. He was smiling.

Once I was transferred from the gurney to the hospital bed, he and his entourage stepped closer. He looked at my neck, listened to my heart, checked my ankles, and introduced himself.

"My name is Dr. Tallaj." It sounded like "collage," except with a "t." I found out later that he was from the Dominican Republic and that his ever-present grin was something of a trademark.

As I shook his hand, he began, "Mr. Burcham, your friends Dr. Drenning and Dr. Allison said you were in pretty bad shape, and looking at you, I agree. A few hours ago, Dr. Drenning recorded heart pressures and outputs 'incompatible' with life—he actually didn't think your heart would last for the trip down here. I ordered him to start you on two intravenous inotropes and a diuretic. We have a team in the operating room waiting to install an LVAD, a left ventricular assist device, in your chest. It's a pump that works in parallel with your own heart, sustaining you until you can be evaluated and listed for a heart transplant. You seem to have improved a bit on the flight down. Do you want to proceed with the procedure or wait and see?"

It was a lot to take in at once. Fortunately, Cindy and Anna burst into the room at that moment, looking frantic and frazzled. Evidently, the transportation mess up in Huntsville and longer flight against headwinds had given them enough time to drive here. Cindy rushed over and grabbed my hand. I gave her a reassuring squeeze and realized that I was very glad I hadn't been sedated for the trip. I might not have been in any shape to have this conversation and participate in the action plan.

"Dr. Tallaj, will you have to crack my chest open to install the LVAD? And then crack it open again when a donor heart is available?" I asked.

"Yes," he nodded. "That's right. Two trips through the operating room, two rough recovery periods."

Looking up at Cindy and Anna, I suddenly felt calm, and the familiar, inaudible presence of the Lord helped me say confidently, "Let's wait and see."

Dr. Tallaj nodded again. "OK, we are going to step out into the hallway, have a team meeting and devise a plan for you. Your nurse, Laura, will be monitoring and administering our orders all night." As an afterthought, he added, smiling, "By the way, Dr. Allison did his internship here with me."

"My neighbor and favorite electrophysiologist interned here?" I said.

"Oh, he's your neighbor? That's convenient. Yes, he did study and practice here." He added more seriously, "You are in very critical condition right now, but we can help you. It's a good thing you were in the care of two former UAB colleagues. I'll see you first thing in the morning."

The Saturday and Sunday following my helicopter ride passed as if I were in a fog. Visitors came and went, but I can't remember who they were, when they stopped by or what they said. Shift after shift, nurses came and went, but I don't remember which ones attended to me. While I was sleeping, Anna used her cell phone to take a short video clip of the distended veins still bulging in my neck 36 hours after my admission. When she showed it to me, I realized why it had been a lot scarier for Cindy than for me that afternoon in Huntsville.

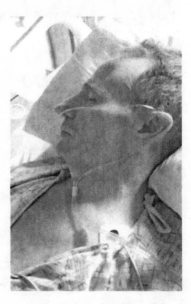

I suppose, not being fully in command of my faculties was a blessing. I didn't have the time or awareness to get frightened about what was happening to me or to become anxious about my future prospects.

Distended veins above the tag

However muddle-headed I may have been, I did have a clear understanding, though, of the treatment plan Dr. Tallaj and his team had laid out for me. They were taking a three-pronged approach to stabilizing me. They were drying me out—less fluid pressing on my organs meant less work for my weak heart.

At the same time, they were reducing my blood pressure to the lowest asymptomatic level possible via oral medications. Finally, they were strengthening my heart muscle through the continued use of intravenous inotropes. (By then, I had had someone explain to me that inotropes were drugs that boosted muscular contractions, which would improve the pumping ability of my heart.)

On a parallel track, a host of physicians and nurses were analyzing my mental and physical capacities with the goal of qualifying me for a heart transplant, the step of last resort for someone in my condition. I hadn't fully come to grips yet with the idea of removing and replacing my heart with a donor heart. I continued to hope for another path forward, while undergoing the battery of tests and meetings.

When I started to feel better and became more lucid, Cindy and I had a conversation about the options: waiting in the hope that my heart would simply get better with treatment or moving forward to a heart transplant. True to my optimistic nature, I argued for the former. Cindy all but read me the riot act. "Steve, you've been on this health roller coaster for over three years now. Whenever you begin to feel well, you conveniently forget you've got heart problems, but I'm the one seeing and dealing with the fallout. If the doctors are convinced you need a heart transplant, then you are getting one!"

Seeing the tears well up in her eyes as she argued the case with fierce passion, I acquiesced.

When I told the doctors of our decision, they said that they anticipated the qualification process would take a week to 10 days.

This brought up an issue regarding Lindsey and Jay's wedding in December. When I learned that, right after I was transferred to UAB, Cindy and Lindsey had the stationery designer make postcards cancelling the wedding, I nearly came unglued. I called my daughter and my future son-in-law to my bedside for a private consultation, and after some discussion and prayers, insisted that "the show must go on!" Cindy, Lindsey and Jay reluctantly agreed. Fortunately, they hadn't yet mailed the postcards and only cancelled the reception hall. That would present a big challenge to Lindsey—to find another venue in short order during the holiday season—but I knew she would be up to it.

As far as my attending the ceremony, the "best-case scenario" the doctors agreed to as a possibility was that I might leave the hospital on oral medications and one intravenous drug if I were still waiting for a donor heart at that point. Depending on one intravenous med would put me near the top of the priority list for heart transplants at status level 1B. The highest priority for patients waiting was 1A, reserved for those too ill to leave the hospital. The lower active status was 2, for those who were stable and ambulatory on oral medications. Status 7 indicated that a patient had been de-listed for some reason.

By the end of the first weekend, I started to feel better and more alert, and felt ready to communicate with the outside world again.

The moment he had heard about my deteriorating health and transfer to UAB, my boss and good friend, Danny Windham, had set up a CaringBridge blog site on my behalf. It allowed me to create a web journal which would apprise others of my condition. When he called to tell me about it, he reported that within two days of my slipping into cardiogenic shock, there were almost 5,000 guest hits on the website. Amazed at the volume of interest, I decided to make the theme of my journal posts more about the *process* of coping with my crisis than the crisis itself. In other words, I would write about my approach to dealing with my health journey. After all, the good Lord had gotten me this far, so I was confident He'd see me through the rest of the way. I mused that if I eventually wrote a book about this crazy adventure of mine, I might call it, *It's Not About My Heart*.

Reflecting on the last few days, I wrote and posted my first CaringBridge journal entry:

> *"This is the first time since I arrived on Friday night that I've felt well enough to sit up and provide an update. Reading your visitor posts brings warm feelings of grace and tears of joy. With friends, colleagues, and family like you, the medical team here at UAB and the gracious healing power of our Lord Jesus Christ, I know I'm in good hands with no worries.*
>
> *As everyone knows by now, on Friday night, I was voted 'most likely to receive an LVAD' by the University's medical team. I began to respond favorably to the medications and we took the decision to wait and see... so avoiding one trip through the operating room is desirable to me. Things can change quickly, so let's continue to pray that I remain stable and improving."*

In the meantime, I felt as well cared for as I had ever experienced. That was a good thing, because I was told that after transplant, the Heart Transplant Intensive Care Unit (HTICU) at UAB would be my clinic for the rest of my life. Have a broken leg? Get the situation stabilized locally and then hightail it here for follow-up care. Sick with a virus or flu? Count on coming in for a visit. Can't hold any food down for some reason? We'll leave the lights on for you here at the HTICU. As one of the doctors told me, "We have seen it all. Need marriage counseling? No problem!"

Considering how close I was to complete heart failure, I was amazed how well I now felt. There was no pain, no CHF symptoms—I wasn't coughing uncontrollably, feeling dizzy or experiencing shortness of breath—and I was able to sleep lying down, something I hadn't been able to do since late spring.

As I settled into the hospital routine, my biological clock refused to adjust, however. I continued to wake up daily between 5:30 and 5:45 a.m. At that time the room was lit only by the glow of the monitoring equipment screens. Since I wouldn't be able to order breakfast for another hour, I would start to get ready for the day by inclining my bed into more of a chair configuration. The city outside the window was faintly visible in the early morning light, and the dull hum of commuter traffic gradually got louder as more and more people made their way to work.

There were several devices I was hooked up to that prevented me from getting up. The heart monitor with four pads stuck to my chest had a wireless computer that fit nicely into my gown's pocket. The peripherally inserted central catheter, or PICC line, entered into a vein right below my right bicep. It had two ports, one for drawing blood and the other for administering intravenous medications. The plastic line inside me was actually about 18 inches long, running from the ports to a discharge point directly above my heart in the blood-intake zone.

From what the nurses told me, I understood that having a PICC line was both a curse and a blessing. On the upside, it allowed the nurses to draw vials of blood for the daily labs without having to stick me over and over again. Also, the drugs I was getting were so powerful that they'd have been too rough on smaller veins, rendering a standard intravenous line useless after a day or two. On the downside, PICC lines and ports had to be well cared for. To prevent infections the waterproof dressing had to be changed often, the entry point had to stay dry at all times, and the access ports dangling from my bicep required daily flushing with both saline solution and heparin, an anticoagulant. Eventually, Cindy and I would be taught to do all that ourselves because for long-term treatment, a PICC line was the way to go. I could have mine for some time while waiting for a donor heart. One nurse told me about another patient of hers who had his PICC line for two years while waiting for a good organ match.

On the Wednesday morning before Thanksgiving, I was looking forward to having the Foley catheter removed, which led from under the blankets to a urine collection bag hooked to the rail of the bed. That would give me mobility for the first time since Friday night when I had been admitted. Considering that I was only going to have a 30-minute procedure in Huntsville and that five days had lapsed before I could go to the bathroom on my own again, the Foley had been a good call, I thought.

The doctors had told me they want me up and walking around the unit. There was a metered track in the hallways of the HTICU: 20 laps equaled one mile. My initial goal would be five laps or one-quarter of a mile. Of course, the intravenous medication hanging on a pole with a wheel base would have to accompany me.

During one of his visits, my boss, who had fought and won a battle with leukemia 15 years earlier, had given me a stuffed monkey named Mickey who was now hanging on my IV pole, "monitoring" the medications. Someone had bestowed Mickey on him back then, and he asked that once I had completed my journey successfully, I pass him along to another patient. I imagined what a conversation piece Mickey would make with his goofy grin, beady eyes and long arms as I'd make my rounds in the unit. I smiled and picked up my daily devotional and decided to have some quiet time before I ordered my breakfast.

Over the last few days, my boss and Brother John had arranged activities back home in support of my recovery. On Monday evening, members of our church and employees of Digium gathered at the Storehouse on Asbury's campus to pray for me. The Storehouse had been set up in the church's original Fellowship Hall as a 24/7 prayer ministry, and I was deeply moved watching a short video clip of the event afterward, seeing so many friends and colleagues petitioning the Lord on my behalf. Brother John had also arranged a daily "prayer time" in a conference room at Digium during the lunch hour. I understand that on the first day about a dozen employees from all denominations came together to lift up my situation to the Lord. I was planning to surprise them by calling into the conference room later in the week and participating in their prayers.

When the catheter was removed, I couldn't wait to get out of bed. I easily completed my laps in the unit to meet my goal. My legs felt a little weak at first, but it wasn't long before I was motoring up and down the hallway quite nicely. When the nurses started weighing me on more accurate scales three days earlier, it turned out that I was only five pounds above my optimal college graduation weight. I joked that I should patent the non-lethal aspects of the diet and drug regimen as "The 20th Reunion Heart Diet—guaranteed to work in 30 days or less."

Best of all, I was not experiencing any CHF symptoms!

Unfortunately, that wasn't good enough to send me home for Thanksgiving. Although I had completed all the tests and evaluations for a heart transplant, I still had to be weaned from the powerful cocktail of intravenous drugs and be sure my diet and activities wouldn't destabilize me. There was also the matter of one final biopsy of my right lung. I had had a couple of nodules there for years, but a new one popped up recently causing some concern among members of the transplant team. They wanted to test it for malignancy.

So I spent the long Thanksgiving weekend in bed, enjoying visits from family and friends and watching a number of football games, including the drubbing Auburn suffered at the hands of the Crimson Tide in the Iron Bowl.

By the weekend, my morning routine had changed to getting coffee, taking some quiet time—the nurses were on two-hour rounds throughout the night—showering, shaving, getting dressed, doing some laps and finishing with breakfast. The morning I managed to walk one and three quarters of a mile without having any issues, Dr. Tallaj happened to be in the unit on an emergency call and saw me fully dressed, doing laps in the HTICU while everyone else was still in bed. When he asked me about the Iron Bowl, grinning—he knew my favorite team had lost—I could honestly tell him, "That was the worst four hours I had all week."

Later in the day, he concluded that I was now "too well" for the HTICU, so I was kicked out and transferred to a regular recovery room on the sixth floor. After the move, I was in bed reading when I felt a flutter in my heart for about ten seconds. It passed and the nurse came by about five minutes later, asking how I felt—my monitoring screen at the nurses' station had triggered an alarm. I had gone into ventricular tachycardia

(V-tach) and the pacemaker that Dr. Allison had installed in October had done its job, remedying the situation without having to deliver a shock.

"That little device has more than paid for itself," I thought.

The doctor who later reviewed the event via computer agreed that it had been routine. There was no reason to be concerned.

On the other hand, I had begun to run a fever, and that was worrisome. My temperature usually ran between 97 and 98 degrees, a little on the low side of normal, but now it was going up as high as 102.8. A week of intravenous antibiotics did not bring it down, and the members of the infectious disease team had been unable to determine the root cause. Just as during my bout with pericarditis in 2009, every culture and test they ran came back with the same result—negative!

With the right lung biopsy completed and the doctors continuing to try to get my fever under control, another week passed. On Friday morning, December 2, Dr. Salpy Pamboukian, a cardiologist working with Dr. Tallaj, stopped by to give Cindy and me an update. She had become the doctor in charge of my case who oversaw my treatment on a regular basis. Of Armenian heritage, she had grown up in Canada before doing her medical schooling in Chicago. She was a striking woman, slender and tall who cared about her appearance and was always dressed to the nines. She actually traveled to Canada by plane from time to time to visit friends and get her hair done! At the same time, she was a no-nonsense, "by the book" professional. She would tolerate kidding around but didn't usually participate and would not budge an inch on anything related to proper patient care. She was definitely the alpha female in the department.

She told us that the heart transplant team had met to discuss my case, and I had been cleared for listing, but wouldn't be put on a list for a donor heart right away. Because I had responded so well to treatment, looking at all the data, the team members were only 70% convinced that I needed a new heart right then. If I were listed, chances I would be getting a new donor heart quickly were high because there were only a few patients in the queue ahead of me, and my B positive blood type allowed me to accept an organ from O blood type donors, which are very common. The bottom line was that because a transplant is a serious undertaking, they wanted me to hang on to my own heart for as long as possible.

"Now you have heart symptoms, but no rejection problems and only minor medication side effects, but with a heart transplant you're essentially trading one set of challenges for another, hoping for an improved quality of life in the bargain," she said.

Her explanation made sense to Cindy and me.

"So what's the plan?" I asked.

Dr. Pamboukian explained that as soon as my fever was under control, I was going to be released from the hospital. I would continue to be on inotrope medication, which would be administered via an electronic intravenous pump that I could wear on my belt. After two or three weeks, I'd return to UAB for a right heart catheterization and to have my heart pressures and pumping efficiency rechecked. Depending on the results, at that point I would either get listed for a heart transplant or continue as before.

That evening, anticipating leaving the hospital soon, I updated my friends and family on CaringBridge and thanked them for their extraordinary efforts:

Your daily guestbook visits to my website bring laughter and tears of joy; they are so uplifting and inspiring. It's good to hear from former Chrysler colleagues, former Siemens and Continental colleagues, the Digium family, the Asbury Family, Fathom youth, Madison & Metro Huntsville area friends, former bosses, family and extended family, Leadership Twenty-One graduates, former Sunday school friends, suppliers, customers, and people I have never had the opportunity to meet!

You are all ministering to me in my time of need. Without you, I think it would be easy to 'drive myself into the ditch' and begin feeling sorry for myself, but that hasn't happened. I want you to know that my family and I are truly blessed to have friends like you!

Through this, I've really learned this time that I simply must let go and let God work through all of you, the caregivers and the experts.

Needless to say, it was easier to write these words than follow them. Despite my best intentions, I grew stir crazy because it took another week before my fever finally disappeared. The doctors never figured out what caused it. I'm convinced I caught a virus while I was laid up in the hospital, and it simply had to run its course.

By the morning of December 8, my temperature had been back to normal for 24 hours. In an effort to send me home only on oral medications, the doctors also weaned me completely off the intravenous inotrope medication without adverse side effects. So at 7 a.m., I was first in line in the catheterization lab to have my heart checked to see how it was doing on its own.

Later, Dr. Pamboukian stopped by with the results, which were mixed. Based on my weight and body size, the team was looking for an overall cardiac output of 2.2. While I was much improved, I still managed to reach only 1.8. I knew the number was accurate because the doctors in the lab got that same reading three times, and I overheard them discussing the results with one another.

The team wasn't comfortable sending me out of the hospital without some extra support for my heart—so much for leaving UAB without an IV pump—and we were back to plan A. The doctors would reinstall the PICC line—they had pulled the original one thinking it had gotten infected, causing the fever—and would start me on Milrinone, a cousin of the medications I had been taking. Milrinone would help the left ventricle of my heart muscle squeeze more forcibly and dilate my blood vessels, dropping my blood pressure so that my cardiovascular system could function at lower stressful levels.

The results of the cardiac output test also left the team 100% convinced that I needed a new heart, and they pronounced me ready to be listed. Dr. Pamboukian agreed to comply with our wishes and wait until after Lindsey's wedding before putting me on the list. Since we were on again after the panicky cancellation in November, we didn't want to get ready for the ceremony, only to receive a call from my transplant coordinator as Lindsey was walking down the aisle, informing us that a donor heart was available.

Remarkably, the day after I told Lindsey, "The wedding must go on," she and Carole were on their way to check out one of the only remaining unbooked venues in Huntsville for the holidays, the North Hall in the Von Braun Center. As they headed toward downtown on I-565, Carole on a hunch asked Lindsey to pull into the Marriott adjacent to the Space and Rocket Center.

Inquiring inside, they learned that a cancellation had occurred just the evening before, which had freed up the Grand Ballroom, and they booked it on the spot for the wedding reception.

All things considered, I figured it would take a small act of Congress to get me out of the hospital by Friday, what with the installation of the PICC line, titrating the new medication to the correct dosage level, ordering a portable intravenous medication pump, teaching me and Cindy how to use it and ensuring that I was stable and OK to go home. I had some sense of what prisoners must feel when their release date approaches. Time slows to an agonizing crawl and the anticipation of freedom is almost unbearable.

But the staff at UAB pulled off a miracle. Working feverishly, the PICC nurses set a new record for getting a patient up to speed—it normally took up to two days; in my case, less than two and a half hours! After everything was installed and properly calibrated, I walked a mile in the unit on the new medication without any problems. The Milrinone dropped my blood pressure into the 80s over 50s range, which was a little unnerving, until the doctors said it was fine as long as I were symptom-free. When they told me to pay attention to my symptoms, not to the numbers, I couldn't resists reminding them that I was an engineer by profession.

Finally, all that remained was to get the portable intravenous medication pump so Cindy and I could get a crash course on how to operate it. With discharge papers in hand and suitcases, backpack, two full baskets of goodies and flower arrangements all stored on a cart next to the bed, we waited in my room for the delivery man to bring the pump and custom mixed medication from the manufacturer across town. Cindy managed to relax in a chair, reading on her Kindle. I, on the other hand, was pacing the floor.

"Where could he be?" I asked repeatedly.

"Steve, relax, they said he was on his way 45 minutes ago. He'll be here soon. Just sit down and take it easy," Cindy said, trying to comfort me.

It was like throwing gasoline on a fire. "Twenty-one days! Nine to stabilize me after cardiogenic shock and twelve for that darn fever to run its course!" I fulminated.

"Yes, but if it were not for that fever, they wouldn't have tried weaning you and checking your heart function one final time."

"Yep, you are right," I conceded. "That little fever allowed the team time to execute a plan that ultimately convinced them I should be listed. I'm just not sure *I* need or want to be listed."

"Steve, stop it. We've already had this discussion. The doctors wouldn't list you if they didn't think it was your only way out— they don't haphazardly give out donor organs, you nut."

About that time, a short, slightly overweight man entered the room. He was a little out of breath and there were sweat stains on his company logo golf shirt. Handing me a cold pack, he said, "Here are your medications. Sorry it took me so long, I had another delivery across town; got here as quickly as I could." He added, "I bet you are ready to bust out of here."

He had no idea!

A short while later, Cindy and I finally left the hospital—on my own steam...no wheelchair this time—three weeks to the day I had entered it clinging to dear life.

Chapter 7
Respite

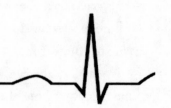

The homecoming was sheer pleasure. On my first evening back, Cindy, Anna and I watched our favorite Christmas movie, "How the Grinch Stole Christmas." That Saturday, I met my home health-care nurse, a friendly woman named Tish who had 16 years of experience as a cardiac nurse and told me that, from now on, we would be like family.

On Sunday, we returned to Asbury for the traditional morning service, and I received a warm reception and lots of hugs and handshakes. It was wonderful to be back in worship service and to see all of our friends who had been so supportive.

I slept very well over the weekend and experienced no negative symptoms whatsoever; I was really looking forward to going back to work on Monday. During lunchtime at Digium, I attended the prayer session that Brother John and my boss, Danny, had scheduled. I enjoyed the opportunity to pray in person with my friends and colleagues who had been praying diligently for me and my family. I put in half a day and spent the rest of the afternoon in my home office. I kept to that schedule for the rest of the week, feeling more confident every day. On Friday, when we held our holiday lunch, we agreed that I would give the invocation. I chose as my theme, "Take nothing for granted this holiday season." I decided to put in at least three full days at work the following week and to be back full-time by the beginning of January.

Capping the week was the wedding of my daughter, Lindsey Morgan Burcham, to Jay Robert Sterling Riffel. Not only did I have the stamina to run errands and attend the rehearsal dinner and make a well received speech there, I survived a long photo session and managed to keep my nerves under control before walking the bride down the aisle.

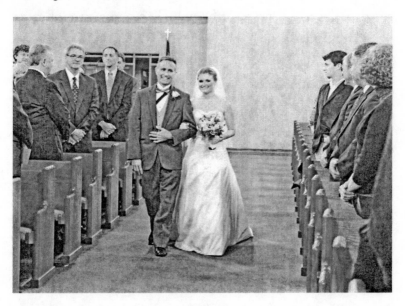

Proud Dad!

Brother John surprised us all when he turned to me and said, "Boy, I sure am glad to see *you* here!" The entire sanctuary erupted in laughter setting a more relaxed tone for the ceremony. Afterward, I enjoyed the reception, which went until 11 p.m., and had a fine time all around. I think I hugged more people than the bride and groom did. By the end of the evening my heart was fine, and my feet were killing me.

I felt flushed with pride seeing my oldest daughter get married, and pleased that I was able to be there for her throughout the weekend. On our way to the wedding ceremony, I even managed to remove a heel-sized dirt stain from her train with my saliva-covered finger—I had heard it said once that a parent's spit is as good as Formula 409 at removing stains, and it turned out to be true. Considering how touch-and-go my life had been just a few weeks ago, I was truly blessed. When I finally relaxed after it was all over, I felt wonderful and almost in a state of grace. Recalling one of my favorite verses from Proverbs (14:30), "A heart at peace gives life to the body," I gave silent thanks to the Lord for allowing me to have this experience.

The following Wednesday, Cindy and I made a trip to the Kirklin Clinic at UAB for a routine visit. It took longer to register than it did to get the blood samples pulled and to see Dr. Pamboukian for my checkup.

Cindy had decided that while we were in Birmingham, we would finish our Christmas shopping. We went to the Homewood section of town, where lots of specialty shops lined the streets. I was thankful that she hadn't included going to the mall in her plans—it's exhausting to get dragged from store to store when you couldn't care less about what most of them have to offer. So, after my visit with the doctor, we headed out, parked in a public lot, went to a small diner for lunch, shopped for a while and decided it was time to head to the SUV before continuing our shopping. By now, the weather had turned sunny and warm. It was almost 70 degrees outside.

The previous evening, while sitting in my easy chair watching television, I had checked my pump and noted that it would run out of intravenous medication by the afternoon of the next day. I told Cindy that we'd have to take everything we needed with us and when it was time to change the medication, return to the SUV and start a new bag.

As we approached our car with gift bags in hand, I noticed two male parking lot attendants were outside their booth leaning against the brick wall not far from us. They were smoking and enjoying the nice weather. Cindy and I opened the tailgate, threw the gifts in the back and then proceeded to get in the backseat of the SUV to reload my medication, swap the pump batteries and flush the PICC lines. In order to complete these tasks, I had to take both my shirt and undershirt off. It took about 10 minutes. When we were done, I started to wrestle with my shirt to put it back on and quickly realized there was no way to tuck it in sitting in the backseat. So I opened the door, got out, tucked in my shirt, zipped up my jeans, buckled my belt and threw on my backpack containing the new bag and pump. As I looked up, I noticed the two guys staring in our direction. At that point, Cindy popped out on the other side of the SUV, straightening her blouse and hair.

We didn't even try to convince the onlookers that we had a legitimate reason for our activities in the backseat. We locked the car, giggled like teenagers and headed back to the stores!

We were still in high spirits when we returned to the clinic to find out the results of the blood tests. The transplant coordinator told me that the labs were complete. Everything was in order and I had been put on the list for a heart transplant with status 1B. When I asked her how long it would take to find a match, she gave me an answer that I adapted for my own use for equally inquisitive friends and family members: "Based on your blood type, you'll go fast."

I continued to feel great. The only difficulty was that about two and a half hours after I took my oral medications, I would have a little "sinking spell." It would last between five and 30 minutes, and I'd have to take it easy during that time. I certainly couldn't bend down and stand up quickly. At some point, I took my blood pressure when it happened and discovered that it was 74 over 45—a drop from my normal 105 over 64. I decided that it was my body's reaction to the drug I was taking and that I'd simply have to manage my way through it.

It turns out that most people have considerably more trouble on Milrinone, and I was fortunate that I had only this one side effect. My nurse gave me a tip for dealing with the "sinking spells"—she told me to sit on the couch, elevate my feet and sip some Gatorade. That worked remarkably well. I always felt much better when I got back up and started moving around the house again.

During the four days between the Christmas holidays and the New Year's weekend, I worked at Digium full-time, completing year-end reports and generating my group's business plan for 2012.

From a health standpoint, I was continuing to do better and better. Three times that week, I went to the gym and walked or jogged on the treadmill. Overall, I logged five and a half miles, two thirds at a fast walk pace and the rest jogging at a 10-minute-mile pace. I knew that for serious runners that was just a stroll in the park, but for me, it was impressive. I hadn't been able to do anything close to it since springtime. For the first time in months, I felt revitalized after exercising.

The highlight of the week was another wedding. Buddy's daughter Laura and her beau, Tommy, got married on New Year's Eve. Laura had been like a sister to my daughters and sometimes called me her "alternate dad." Lindsey and Jay had stayed in town for the event before heading back to Houston, but our middle daughter, Brooke, could not attend—she was in Sydney, Australia with a group from Auburn's Building Science department. The ceremony turned out to be another glorious union of a beautiful bride and handsome groom at Asbury with Brother John again performing the service.

The reception was held at the Huntsville Museum of Art downtown and the party went well beyond midnight. Cindy kept a close eye on "her heart patient," allowing my friend, David, to sneak me only one cocktail during the course of the evening and just a single glass of champagne at midnight. Following the New Year's toast and kisses, we all filed outside into the chilly air. Under the glow of city lights brightened by occasional flashes of fireworks, we lined the circular driveway entrance to the museum, holding giant sparklers. It was another enchanted moment for the new couple and all attending the wedding.

As I woke up the next morning, I felt the best I had ever felt on New Year's Day—no headache, no heart symptoms, a bright new year ahead.

I'd made it an annual ritual to make my New Year's resolutions that day. I was happy to note that I had achieved 13 of my 15 objectives for 2011. The one I'd penned a year earlier about my health was, "Take heart condition seriously—diet, take medications, follow doctor's orders, seek to find answers." Even though the answers remained elusive, I decided that I had given it a yeoman's effort!

As I sat down to generate my list for 2012, I was determined to make no allowances for my condition. I would not put my life on hold, or let any fears and doubts become part of the journey I was undertaking. I intended to faithfully and confidently engage in the process and proceeded to plan ahead just as in any normal year.

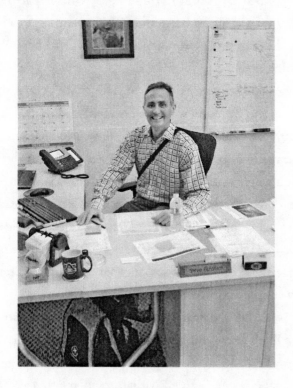

Working at Digium,
pump at my side

Chapter 8
Close Call

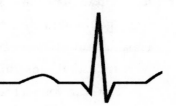

My resolutions were put to the test the following morning when I emerged from deep sleep into dim awareness that Cindy was shaking me, saying, "Steve! Steve! Wake up, your cell phone is ringing, you must get it." The urgency in her voice intermingled with the soft musical ringtone issuing from the kitchen counter-top where I park my phone for charging each night.

I unpeeled myself from the sheets, picked up the Milrinone pump in its satchel and headed for the kitchen, but by the time I got there, the ringing had stopped.

Immediately, Cindy's cell phone started up in her office adjacent to the dining room.

"It must be one of the kids, an emergency of some sort. Hurry!" she called out to me.

"It's the UAB heart transplant team," I called back. "They left a message on my phone."

Then another ringing sound resonated through the house— our landline. This time I picked it up in time. It was one of the on-call transplant coordinators. She informed me that a donor heart had become available, and put me on "standby" status; I was to sit tight here in Madison and await a call back within three hours with more instructions.

As I hung up, I glanced at the clock on the desk. The digital display read 3:30 a.m. Considering the alarming intrusion into our nighttime slumber and the momentousness of the news, I remained surprisingly unaffected. I simply caught Cindy up on what the coordinator had told me and headed back to bed.

"How can you go back to sleep knowing it's finally going to happen?" she asked, incredulous.

"Because I'm tired, that's how," I replied.

But Cindy wouldn't have it. "You are *not* going back to bed," she insisted. "We are getting up and getting ready. Go put on some coffee."

By the time the aroma of freshly brewed coffee dripping into the carafe filled the kitchen, I was fully awake. I decided it was time to have "the talk" with Cindy, but I knew I would have to wait until she had at least half a cup of joe in her. Unlike me, she is not a morning person.

It was 4:30 a.m. when she came into my study. She had showered and dressed and was in full "nesting mode." She had gotten cleaning supplies out and was running the flat mop around the hardwood floors on the main level of the house. Then she attacked the upstairs. The last time I'd seen her behaving like this had been 23 years earlier when she was expecting Lindsey. She had awakened me in the middle of the night then, too, and informed me that this was the day, but allowed me to go back to sleep while she cleaned our three-bedroom, two-bathroom house from bow to stern. Then she had barged into our bedroom and announced, "Get up, breakfast is ready and the coffee is on. Eat, and then let's go to the hospital."

Which is just what we did.

It was a dark, moonless night. I remembered seeing a bright shooting star over downtown Huntsville, and I felt calm and peaceful, certain that everything was going to be OK. Some hours later, Lindsey came into the world, a healthy, seven-pound, two-ounce baby girl. For some reason, I started to cook breakfast for our family the day after she came home, and have done so ever since.

When Cindy finally joined me in my study, looking a bit haggard, I asked her to sit down. I showed her the file whose contents I had been looking over and pulled out a one-page information sheet I had put together for my family. On the front side was a spreadsheet itemizing our assets, bank accounts, insurance policy info and other financial records. On the back were instructions for my funeral service. I went as far as listing my favorite scripture verses, songs and who I wanted to sing them. Although I worshipped "traditionally" every Sunday, I wanted an upbeat "celebration of life" at Asbury's Grace Building, with rock praise bands and all.

"This paper here has everything you need to know on it," I explained. "If something goes wrong, just get with Buddy, and he'll help you execute this plan. Pay off the house, put the rest into safe investments, and you'll be set."

"Nothing's going to go wrong," she said grumpily.

Undeterred, I continued to talk to her about a "do not resuscitate" order and other medical decisions she might have to make. "If I'm comatose and not responding to treatment, use biblically significant numbers to guide your decisions. For example, if the doctor suggests we should see some improvement in a week to ten days, give it seven for healing and prayer to work and then pull the plug. I don't want to be on endless life support draining everyone's energy and our resources. OK?"

Cindy gave me an indulgent look. "Thanks for sharing your thoughts with me, but nothing's going to go wrong!" She stood up abruptly and exited the study to perform more cleaning tasks.

Two hours later, we finally got our second call. The instructions were simple and straightforward: Report to Birmingham as soon as possible. It felt so routine and unreal at the same time, I decided not to notify anyone else about what was happening yet.

It was a cool, sunny day. We headed to the UAB, with me at the wheel of our SUV. At some point, I looked over at Cindy and said, "This is not 'it,' is it? False alarm. I just feel it."

"Me too, I don't believe it's time either," Cindy agreed.

When we arrived in the ambulatory cardiothoracic (ACT) room at the HTICU, there were three other patients already being prepped as potential organ recipients. Nurses were busy checking their vitals, logging results in computers and trying to keep everyone comfortable.

The nurse that greeted me, Laura—I referred to her as "little Laura"—was young, sweet, bubbly and always in a cheerful mood. "Well, that was fast Mr. Burcham. You've only been home a few weeks, and now you get to be my first heart transplant work-up," she said with a smile and pointed to a leather chair in the corner waiting for me.

Because of my history of lung nodules, as part of the intake the doctors sent me down to the lab for a CT scan, which revealed that a few more had popped up. They were smaller than the tip of a pencil, but raised enough concern to have me taken off the transplant list—I was officially de-listed at status 7—until they could be investigated further and ruled harmless. The heart transplant team wanted to get to the bottom of the lung issue quickly and planned to schedule me for appointments with three physicians—cardio, pulmonary and infectious disease.

Two hours after our arrival, Cindy and I were back in the car heading home.

I felt fine about it. With no pulmonary symptoms whatsoever, I wasn't worried about my lungs. I figured going through the motions would prove me right and hopefully allow me some time to get more comfortable with the idea of receiving a new heart, and the fact that someone else would have to die so that I could go on living. Despite all the activity and conversations about it with the transplant team, I still couldn't wrap my head around it.

The next day Cindy and I returned to UAB for my regular appointment with Dr. Pamboukian, who had sprung into action quickly. As a follow-up to my heart transplant dry run, she had scheduled me for a PET scan, a meeting with an infectious disease doctor and a meeting with a thoracic surgeon for the following day. She also scolded me for jogging on the treadmill last week. "Walking fast is OK but jogging or running is *not* OK."

Having the PET scan done and the results evaluated took all day. The good news was that neither the old nor the new lung nodules lit up and therefore no longer concerned the infectious disease doctor. The two enlarged lymph nodes that showed up next to my heart, however, did. The transplant team wanted to take a closer look and scheduled a biopsy for the following week. The understandable concern was that if I had an infection of any kind, it could spread through my body after the heart transplant because my immune system would be suppressed.

I tried to find meaning in the frustrating runaround. It was almost as if the Lord were drawing out the process so that I could work on a Christian character trait that had always been difficult for me to grasp, let alone practice: namely, surrender—the relinquishment of one's own will to a higher power. Each time I'd heard about it from the pulpit or in a study group, I said to myself, "It's time to start working on that—surrendering, really, really letting go and allowing God to work." But more times than not, I'd prayed and laid a problem at the feet of our Lord, only to take it back the next day; as if I could fix it better than He!

One afternoon in my office at Digium, it really dawned on me: I did not have control over *anything*. I didn't know when I would be ready, really ready, to receive a heart—I continued to struggle with the idea of someone else's organ inside me—or when a heart would become available for me. I had no idea how long it would take for me to recover from surgery, how long I would be homebound, or when I would be able to go back to work, let alone golf or fish.

When I shared these thoughts with my CaringBridge friends, I asked for their prayers to help me to surrender and trust that God's mission for me was far from over. While the journey ahead would be difficult, He would finish the work He had started in me.

Although the following week was not as eventful, it proved no less interesting. Because the procedure to biopsy the lymph nodes near my heart was scheduled for 5:45 a.m. on Tuesday morning, Cindy and I drove to Birmingham after work on Monday in time to grab dinner at the Fish Market Restaurant and watch the BCS National Championship Game in our hotel room at the Residence Inn. Our college football loyalty lies first with Auburn, then Alabama, and after that, to the teams in the SEC, so we really enjoyed watching the Crimson Tide shut out the Louisiana State University Tigers.

The next day was once again mostly about prep and waiting. The biopsy procedure itself was quick and easy. When it was done around 2:30 p.m., I was told that the results would be available by Friday. On the way home, I called family members to let them know I was OK after undergoing surgery. I was confident that nothing serious would show up.

But when we arrived home about three hours later, there was a letter from UAB waiting in the mailbox. We headed inside, and while I went to hang up my coat, I overheard Cindy say, "Well, that's ominous." As I walked into the kitchen, she handed me a "welcome aboard" letter from UAB's Comprehensive Cancer Center with the business card of a "patient navigator" clipped to the upper left hand corner! Not once had I thought the lung nodules were cancerous, but now with "the C word" rattling around in the front lobes of my brain, I was fretting about the results of the biopsy. How was I going to make it to Friday without worrying myself sick?

Fortunately, work at Digium required my undivided attention, and the rest of the week went by quickly. Late on Friday afternoon, Dr. Minnich, the surgeon who had removed the tissue, finally called and informed me that the lymph node biopsy had come back "benign"—no lymphoma or other cancers were detected. He said that the handwringing was over: He was ready to give his go-ahead for a heart transplant to the team. I didn't have much time to rejoice, though, because I soon received another call from Yen, a young transplant coordinator. She just wanted me to know that the team might still want me to see a pulmonologist and that I shouldn't be surprised if I got scheduled for an appointment. The heart transplant "pre-game" show was entering its third week!

But then the team decided it was time to get down to brass tacks and meet with Dr. McGiffin, one of the two heart transplant surgeons at the HTICU. Late Saturday morning, January 14, Cindy and I walked into the waiting room adjacent to those large golden letters on the wall whose message I dreaded every time I passed them. Only one family and another single patient were in the sparsely furnished room. The television was turned to cartoons for kids, and I spent an hour pacing and watching them before Dr. McGiffin himself came in and guided us to a conference room. It looked just like a corporate boardroom with a media player, computer keyboard, conference phones and a giant flat screen monitor on one wall.

As we sat down in unison across from one another, I handed him a file I had generated containing my entire cardiac history. While he reviewed the leading summary sheet and the recounting of events, treatments and diagnoses I'd been through, he asked, "So, how are you doing today?"

"I haven't felt this good in six to nine months," I replied, pulling out my cell phone and waving the photo of me jogging on the treadmill.

Cindy interjected, "Doctor, once he begins to feel better for any stretch of time, he starts minimizing his heart problems and insists that they're 'going to be fine.' It's driving me crazy because I'm living through these highs and lows with him. I'm just ready for him to be better for a good long time."

Dr. McGiffin looked up from my file, fixed his eyes on me over his reading glasses and said, "How many times do you have to be hit over the head before you believe you have a serious heart problem? You might not live through another episode. You need a heart transplant. Now!"

There was a long pause as he turned his stare from me to Cindy and back.

"Yes, sir, I hear you loud and clear," I said sheepishly.

"I will personally clear everything with the team," he continued. "Any more questions?"

We shook our heads.

"The next time I see you will be in the operating room," he said as he collected the papers. Then he stood up and guided us to the door.

That meeting with Dr. McGiffin proved pivotal for me. In mid-November, I had declared to myself, "There's no way in hell I'm going to get a heart transplant," and while Cindy and the doctors had covered a lot of ground regarding my condition, I had only paid lip service to their recommendations and had continued to pray for a different route.

I may not have conveyed in these pages the depths of despair I sometimes felt, but I must admit that I prayed in my chair and on my knees many times, asking, like Jesus in the garden of Gethsemane, for the Father to "take this cup away from me."

Now it seemed inevitable that I must accept the path forward that the Lord had mapped out for me. With Dr. McGiffin delivering a curt message, He had finally gotten through to me. Coming to terms with my pending heart transplant may have been a difficult drink to swallow, but drink this cup I must. "Thy will be done."

On the drive home, I began to wonder out loud how I would have coped with my current situation had it occurred at another time in my life. Reminiscing with Cindy about "where we had been" individually, as a family, and in our spiritual development during the 1980s, 90s and in early 2000, we concluded that it was happening to us now because we were best prepared to deal with it now.

After we finished our conversation, I continued to think about it while I drove and Cindy picked up her reading—she can read without getting carsick. As I reflected more deeply, I came to the realization that I had spent so much time over the last two and a half months trying to find another way around the trip ahead of me, that I hadn't prepared myself all that well for the journey ahead. Yes, I had made some progress mentally and spiritually, but what else should I be doing to get ready?

How does God build our character in preparation for the challenges in our journeys here on earth? I believe one way is through trials and testing. I like the way Peter frames this issue: "In all this you greatly rejoice, though now for a little while you may have had to suffer grief in all kinds of trials. These have come so that the proven genuineness of your faith—of greater worth than gold, which perishes even though refined by fire—may result in praise, glory and honor when Jesus Christ is revealed" (1 Peter 1:6-7).

I certainly felt like I was being refined by fire in the smithy of the Lord. After a few scrapes, I finally came to the realization that there was no need for me to try and change plans because His plans are perfect. I needed to change my perspective, adjust my level of preparedness, trust, believe and allow the rest of His purpose to unfold.

From that point on, I no longer fretted about my trip into uncharted waters. I had complete faith and trust in my guide.

I remember in early February, when Greg, a colleague at Digium, caught me in the hallway and asked, "How do you do this, Steve? How are you staying so calm and upbeat? How do you sleep at night? Aren't you worried?"

Around the same time, another coworker said, "Your faith is so big, how did it get that way? There's no way I'll ever have faith that big or strong!"

Here's what I shared with them and later on included in my CaringBridge post to friends and family:

As far back as I remember I've been blessed with a positive and optimistic view of life. Nonetheless, as a grade-school kid I occasionally had "night frights" during which I dreamed about life ticking by so fast that it would be over before I knew it, and I would be cast into the darkness of space, never to be heard of again. It always was a scary moment waking up after one of those dreams, but in the light of the new day, I would forget about them.

After Cindy and I got married and started raising our kids, I decided that I had spent almost five years learning about science and engineering, and it was time to learn a little more about God. At Asbury, we signed up for disciple classes three years in a row. I have fond memories of going through that first class with the charter members of the church and Pastor Carboni.

As I learned and understood more, I put the "present tense" of eternal life in the bank. I began living out my faith knowing that I possessed eternal life starting the day I believed, not at some point in the future when I died. This was the answer to my childhood nightmares and took care of the "big picture." I started living my life leveraging the power of our faith through the Holy Spirit. I can thrive in the midst of all of this because I know the good Lord has got my back and has my short and long-term needs covered.

When it comes to my behavior, I'm feeling OK and not acting the worried-sick part right now. It's not my nature to lie on the couch, with an ice pack on my heart, waiting for the donor call. I'm not going to change the way I live with faithful optimism because I'm listed for a heart transplant.

After returning from the hospital last week, I did 30 minutes of cardio, and this weekend I plan to finish my early pre-spring yard maintenance. As soon as it warms up again, I'm going to the driving range or I may play the short course with Brooke at Hampton Cove golf course. I'll for sure go fishing with my team at work and hope the telephone call interrupts something fun I'm doing with my friends or family because I don't want to be found fretting my life away because of my heart failure.

I've come to realize that faith is faith—size doesn't matter—and to pray is to be heard and to be heard is to be answered. Our correct response is to believe with childlike confidence, approach tomorrow with childlike wonder, live our lives accordingly and simply amaze Him.

CHAPTER 9

GETTING A NEW HEART

February 12 was a cool, crisp, sunny winter day. I was finishing up my yard maintenance in anticipation of spring, deadheading the Knock Out Roses lining our sidewalk. With the buzzing of the electric trimmer, I must have missed my cell phone ringing and vibrating in my pocket moments earlier. As I began the arduous task of carefully bagging rose trimmings without getting stuck by thorns through my gloves, Cindy appeared on the front porch waving her cell phone at me. The expression on her face made it clear that it was important.

It was Yen from the heart transplant clinic informing me that they had a donor offer. "We are still very early in the process," she said. "Do not rush, but finish whatever you are doing and get down here by 2:00 p.m."

"No problem," I said. "We are only an hour and fifteen minutes away. We can be there by one or one-thirty at the latest."

"Good. I won't see you today but the team will be waiting for you in the HTICU."

An unexpected sense of serenity descended on me when I realized that this was *the* call.

When I calmly told Cindy, she reacted in the same way. Unruffled, she put away her staining supplies, washed out her paintbrushes and started to make some calls. She had been right in the middle of re-staining the oak steps leading from the main floor to the upstairs area of our house. The project had been on our "things to do" list for years.

After I finished bagging the rose trimmings, I put away the wheelbarrow, wound up the extension cord, stashed away the trimmer and rake, and got cleaned up inside.

At some point, Cindy's dad, Ron, stopped by in his Mini to pick up Dixie and her belongings. He looked more panicked than either of us felt. We had to reassure him that there was no reason to panic. We told him we would keep him and Barb in the loop on my progress. After hugging both Cindy and me, he finally gathered up Dixie and her food, toys and blanket, and headed to his house for a stay with their cat, Maxine.

We called Doug and Mary Lou, our neighbors, let them know what was going on and asked them to pick up our mail for us. While driving off, we waved at them as if we were leaving on a vacation.

"This is for real this time, isn't it?" I asked Cindy.

"I've got a good feeling it is, too, Steve. I believe you are going to get a new heart today," she replied confidently.

"I think you are right!"

As we walked into the ACT room in the HTICU, the first thing we noticed was that we were the only ones there! Back in January, other patients and members of their families had occupied the room, hoping they would be the ones receiving the donor organs that day, but this time it was as empty as a church on Tuesday.

As Cindy and I stood there a little dumbfounded, a nurse walked in. She introduced herself as Claire.

"I'll be working you up for a heart transplant today. Exciting isn't it?" she said with a smile as she directed me to a high-backed, leather armchair.

"Where is everybody?" Cindy inquired.

"This is everybody! You've got the room to yourself today. Call your family, hang out and enjoy your company today. You know it's going to be a long 'hurry-up-and-wait' day," Claire said while placing a thermometer in my mouth and taking my pulse.

"The back-up patient for the heart was called off, a bad tissue match," she continued. "You are a perfect match, so if everything goes well, you'll be getting a new heart today, Mr. Burcham."

I flashed back to the first time I had entered this room, when it reminded me of the kidney dialysis center where we used to take G.G., Cindy's grandmother, years ago. It had the same type of armchairs with lots of equipment and gear next to them. The flashback memory was bittersweet. G.G. was an energetic, fun-loving, upbeat Southern lady who had a smile for everyone and always hummed a happy tune, but at 81 she gave up her fight with kidney disease because she didn't want to go through the motions and be a burden to the family. I was frustrated with her decision at the time to go off dialysis, but I didn't know how to convince her otherwise. It only took 20 days before we held a nice service for her.

Cindy's mom, Eve, had a dream about G.G. on the night I was flown to UAB, in which G.G. spoke to me and said, "You're not supposed to be here!" She was more or less "shooing me away" from her in heaven, matching my feelings at the time and now again that my journey here was far from over.

Since false alarm calls are a common occurrence while waiting for a transplant, we had made a pact with our family and friends that we would not notify anyone until we got an official "operating room" time. Simply being called to Birmingham was not enough reason to send out an alert via CaringBridge to energize the prayer team! A few close friends and family members who did not agree with this plan had asked to be put on a "first-call" list and informed directly.

By late afternoon, our neighbors Steve and Traci stopped by; they were in Birmingham already visiting their son Wes. Then Brooke arrived from Auburn and Anna from Orlando. By early evening, Eve appeared with Cindy's sister, Sandra and her husband Stephen; and then my parents showed up shortly after that. We took Nurse Claire's recommendation to heart and rearranged the ACT room, occupying a good half of it with all visitors enjoying their own, personalized leather chairs. For most of the afternoon and evening, we simply sat around, ignored the television and talked. Occasionally, someone would ask me if I were concerned or worried and I invariably replied, "No, not at all." At various times, I nodded off for little naps.

"Lindsey and Jay are looking for puppy hotels in Houston. If we get an OR time, they are planning to pull an all-nighter and drive over," Cindy reported after a cell phone call.

"Nonsense," I said. "Tell them to book direct flights over. I'll pay the fare; I don't want them driving all night!"

"Steve, they checked. Flights that are normally $180 are almost 900 bucks each on short notice."

"I understand, but I'm worried about them driving all night."

Suddenly, Tracy, the nurse who had taken over for Claire at shift change, walked into the room and interrupted our conversation. "The OR is scheduled for 2 a.m. You are a go for a heart transplant!"

Immediately, there was a flurry of activity in the ACT room. Friends and members of my family got busy fishing out their cell phones to text and call others. Anna, as my surrogate CaringBridge correspondent, grabbed the laptop and began to frantically type a quick update. A bevy of nurses descended on me to take more vital sign readings.

Surveying the chaos, Tracy said confidently, "Steve, we are not going to shave you until right before we go to the OR. So after midnight, this place is going to be really crazy! Until then, y'all just try to take it easy, enjoy each other's company and don't worry; everything is going to be fine. Tomorrow you'll be all better!"

I didn't feel any twinges of anxiety, only a low-level sense of being slightly on edge in anticipation of *the* event, but mostly I was glad to be in the presence of people I loved who loved me back and cared for me.

At some point Cindy reported, "Lindsey and Jay found an open-all-night puppy hotel near their airport. They are en route with lots of snacks and energy drinks, and will be here tomorrow morning."

We had been waiting in the ACT room for seven hours, but now the time seemed to pass rather rapidly, and it wasn't long before two male nurses arrived and announced, "Family, it's time to step out. We've got to shave Mr. Burcham from neck to toe, and it's not going to be a pretty sight!"

They were about my height, but broader in the shoulders. One was clean-shaven and looked a bit like Steve Carell. The other looked like a hunter, sporting a closely groomed mustache and beard.

While everyone filed out of the room, the one with the mustache spread a big green sheet on the floor while the other put up freestanding cloth blinds. The employee locker room entrance was on the back wall of the ACT room, so some foot traffic came through from time to time, and I guessed the blind was to prevent a nurse on break from getting flashed by a naked, hairless guy!

After completing their equipment setup and checks, the two nurses huddled up and flipped a coin, much like the team captains do before a football game.

"You got the front, sorry!" clean-shaven said to mustache.

"That's two in a row," mustache complained as he knelt down and started shaving my ankles with an electric razor.

Soon, I was as hairless as a newborn babe. Combined with my weight loss, I was sure I looked like a Sphynx cat standing on that sheet surrounded by little curls of dark fuzz. The nurses spared the hair on my head and taped a tightly fitting surgeon's cap over it instead.

Then I was in the hallway on a gurney, fully prepped and ready to go, operating room doors within reach but closed. Everyone who had spent the day with me in the ACT room stopped by one-by-one for a final hug and kiss. Cindy lingered a little longer, gave me a long kiss and said, "I know everything's going to be just fine." Then she slowly backed away from the gurney, finally releasing my hand as she turned to join the others. I waved at the group as they walked down the long hallway and disappeared into the waiting room.

By now it was early morning on February 13. "Good thing I'm not superstitious," I thought.

As I stared at the drop-tile ceiling, I prayed one last time.

Suddenly, the doors to the operating room flew open.

"Let's go, Mr. Burcham," one of the male nurses said and wheeled me into the brightly lit and freezing OR.

"How are you doing? Are you ready to get a new heart?"

"I'm ready! Let's get this done."

The last thing I remember is a blue mask being fitted over my nose and mouth and the doctor saying, "OK, here goes the anesthesia. See you in a little while..."

Chapter 10

Recovery!

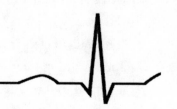

When I came to, I found myself in a dimly lit control room. I could make out operators in scrubs sitting behind consoles and flat screen monitors, looking like they were taking notes and checking data, but I wasn't sure what they were doing. Fighting not to close my eyes, I wondered, "Where am I? Who are these people? What time is it? What day is it?" But I soon drifted off to sleep again...

Sometime later, I came to again. I was determined to stay awake this time and figure out what was going on. I could see others like me lying motionless in adjacent areas of the room. They also had controllers at consoles monitoring them as if they were uranium fuel rods in a nuclear power plant ready to overheat. I decided that the dim illumination in the room came from the overhead lights being switched off with only a patchwork of emergency lights and the glow from monitoring equipment filling the darkness.

I noticed David Letterman on a small television hanging from the ceiling. That meant it was late at night, which didn't make any sense. It had been a little before 4:00 a.m. Monday when I went in for the four-hour surgery to receive a heart transplant.

Everything my senses were telling me just didn't compute, how could Letterman be on television at that hour?

Looking down at my body, I surveyed the myriad tubes and wires that had me pinned down. There were air bladder wraps around the lower parts of my legs that seemed to be on some kind of pre-programmed inflate-deflate cycle. Three tubes that protruded from my midsection were draped over the chrome railing on the left side of the bed and emptied into plastic collection bins. Both of my wrists were equipped with white pads similar to those that rollerbladers wear for protection, except these had tubes coming out of the fingertips that connected to something beyond my field of vision.

I recognized the familiar PICC line inserted under my right bicep. There was also a softball-sized round ball to my right with a tube that connected to somewhere under my gown. While I could not see it, I certainly knew it was there. Two wires issued from my chest, one orange, the other blue—a perfect match of Auburn's school colors, I thought—which were just dangling, not connected to anything. I had a large plastic manifold-like connector protruding from the right side of my neck with lots of tubes hooked up to it and running somewhere out of sight to my right. And finally, I could feel a tube in my throat that allowed me to breathe but limited my head movement and prevented me from talking.

My personal controller must have taken notice of my movements because she suddenly appeared at my side. I motioned for her to change the bed into a more upright sitting position. As she leaned over to push the appropriate buttons to do so, I noticed her nametag—Laura, R.N. I motioned with both of my padded wrists and hands, tubes flying, for her to provide me with a pen and a piece of paper; and then I drifted off to sleep again...

When I woke up the next time, I realized right away that I was in a highly monitored, critical care area of the hospital. Laura, the nurse taking care of me, was still there. She smiled as she handed me a clipboard with a blank piece of paper and a pen. I managed to take hold of the clipboard and place the pen in the upper left-hand corner of the paper before my eyes rolled back in my head—asleep again...

Waking, I saw Laura still waiting by my side. She smiled and handed me the clipboard, which had the word "Wow" written at a negative 45-degree angle and trailing a long, squiggly tail of ink to the bottom of the page. "My first attempt at communicating," I thought.

Concentrating all my strength, I managed to scrape out, barely legibly, "Cough?"

She smiled kindly. "Mr. Burcham, you have a breathing tube in your throat. I have notified the doctors that you have been trying to wake up for about 30 minutes now. They will be here shortly to get it out, I promise."

Writing again, clumsily, I printed, "Good. How long shall I be here?"

"Mr. Burcham, you are doing fine. After the tube is removed, we'll keep you here several more hours to make sure your lungs are functioning well, your oxygen saturation levels are good and your new heart is performing as expected," she said calmly, as I nodded off once more...

When I came to yet again, I picked up the clipboard on my chest right away and started to write. Laura, who had returned to her console, noticed and came over to see what I wanted now.

"Can I see my wife and family?"

"Mr. Burcham, your wife, friends and family already came by. They went to their hotel rooms for rest. You will have to wait until later today to see them again."

Now I was completely confused! When I first woke up, Letterman was on television. Now my family is gone—but already visited with me? When? Why weren't they able to hang around after a four-hour procedure? What was going on?

"Huh?" I wrote.

"Mr. Burcham, it's around 3:00 a.m. Tuesday morning. You've been under anesthesia almost 24 hours," Laura patiently explained. "Your heart transplant went just fine. However, on Monday you experienced heavy internal bleeding all day, and the doctors performed a second emergency surgery last night. Your family saw you right before that surgery and went home three hours later after they learned you were OK and in recovery. They were all up over 36 hours and looked like they needed some shut-eye."

Oh, no! Emergency surgery! The doctors probably scared the daylights out of my wife and daughters, and they had a last minute "viewing of the body" before I went into the OR in case I didn't make it through.

Laura must have read the concern on my face, because she continued reassuringly, "Dr. Melby was very good with your family. He explained that bleeding occurs in about ten percent of these cases and going back in is a fairly routine event. He and the team were glad they did because they were able to fix some things that would have taken much longer to heal on their own."

At that point, a doctor and nurse practitioner arrived to pull out the breathing tube. After some quick coaching and fast, efficient movement on their part, I was able to talk again, dry mouth and all, and respond to their question, "Mr. Burcham, you are looking good. How do you feel?"

"Like I've done a month's worth of yard work in one day," I said. "Let's see, I have a dull headache, my chest is numb and my mouth is dry. Other than that, I feel like getting up!"

Laura brought me a Styrofoam cup of ice water with a straw, which I downed quickly. After she got me a refill, she told me the rest of the story.

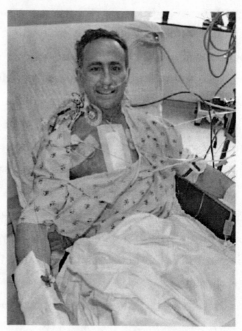

Awake after the heart transplant

As my old heart had gotten weaker, it compensated so much, that over time it expanded to fill every available square inch of space in my chest cavity. When it was removed and a smaller, younger and healthier heart was put in its place, the vacant areas wouldn't heal and stop bleeding, so the doctors decided to open my chest again to locate, stitch and cauterize dozens of small bleeding points on the tissue walls.

While getting me water, Laura must have called into the hospital paging system and announced, "Mr. Burcham is alive, kicking and wants to talk!" After shift change at 7:00 a.m., a steady stream of nurses and doctors stopped by in their street clothes on their way home. They expressed their delight at seeing me sitting up, bright-eyed and bushy-tailed, talking, asking questions and feeling like a new man.

By then a new nurse, who was bubbling with energy, had replaced the more taciturn Laura. She soon wheeled me out of the "control room" into a smaller, private room in the adjacent critical care unit (CCU), informing me that I might be there most of the morning because my room in the HTICU wasn't ready yet; it still needed to be cleaned and sanitized. Then she gave me a bath, washed my hair and dressed me in a fresh gown. It took three nurses to help me from the bed to the chair: one on my left to carry the three catch-bins, another in back of me to keep all the intravenous tubes and monitoring wires from becoming a tangled mess, and the third to steady my balance. But by 9:30 a.m., I was sitting upright in a comfortable recliner ready to receive visitors.

My new nurse was delighted with the results, much like a young girl playing with dolls admiring her work after she had set up a miniature tea party with the participants fully dressed, hair brushed, and ready to play. Considering all that had transpired this morning—waking up with no pain, being alert and talkative, getting cleaned up and out of bed, and being fussed over like a new puppy—I felt an abundance of His grace. I deemed myself blessed beyond measure to simply be alive and was glad to be among these angels taking care of me!

"Hey, look at you! How are you feeling?" Cindy said entering the room. She smiled and came over and gave me a kiss.

Although excited to see me alert, she was not surprised. Apparently, the nurses had already tipped her off that "Chatty Cathy" was sitting up, talking, hassling them with demands for information—the latter from the charge nurse who had the sense of humor of a drill sergeant—and trying to direct the activities in the room: I was thirsty, I was hungry, I was supposed to be recovering in the HTICU. Why couldn't I get any lunch? Why weren't the nurses monitoring my vitals every 15 minutes? I had a new heart in my chest! I'd come a long way; and I certainly wanted to make sure nothing went wrong now, just hours after I woke up! Maybe it was the steroids that put me a little on edge.

Cindy handed me my cell phone and told me to call my dad and then her parents, who had traveled home yesterday and wanted to know how I was doing.

When my dad picked up, I started my conversation as I always do with, "Hey, Pappy, how are you doing?"

There was a brief silence and then, sounding like he was choking back tears, he said, "Son, I can't believe it's you, you sound perfectly normal. This is so unexpected, how do you feel?"

That seemed to be the question of the day. Sara and then Cindy's parents all echoed my dad's surprise. Everyone was amazed that I seemed to be my normal self on the telephone.

The morning in my private little room in CCU went by fast as my three daughters and new son-in-law came by in twos and threes to visit according to the rules, which were being strictly administered by the sergeant-in-charge.

At some point, Dr. Melby came by and delivered the good news that I was doing very well. He also mentioned that the transplant team had determined what had caused my heart failure. It was cardiac sarcoidosis, an autoimmune disease whose fundamental causes were unknown. It tended to present most often itself in the lungs, skin and eyes, and only rarely in other organs such as the heart. Apparently, African-American men, redheaded Irish females and white males of Scandinavian descent are more likely than others to get it. One of the doctors had said that I had the "worst case" the pathologist had ever seen. Another had commented that it was a "most impressive" display of sarcoidosis. (Coincidently, my dad has traced our genealogy back to Denmark circa the 1500s.)

Not that it made any difference anymore, but my doctors now had a clear understanding that my natural heart had been done, and we were unknowingly running out of solutions other than a transplant; and I had a name to put to the root cause of all that I had experienced.

Snapping a photo of me sitting up in the chair looking like I'd had a "wardrobe malfunction" with my gown, Cindy asked Lindsey to post the picture and Dr. Melby's information and progress report as a quick update on CaringBridge.

As my other daughters pointed out that I had gotten a really big present just in time for Valentine's Day, a new heart, an orderly arrived with a gurney at the door and announced that he was here to take me to my room in the HTICU.

Still feeling high, I quipped, "The second present just in time for Valentine's Day: getting out of this closet run by Colonel Klink's twin sister!"

Nurse Tracy met us at the door of Room P539, the "Presidential Suite" in the HTICU, a negative-air-pressure room with a double-door airlock entryway system designated for those who are really sick and can't be swapping germs with everyone else here via the heating, cooling and ventilation systems. While I didn't think I'd need all of the state-of-the-art technology, I was happy to see that the room had huge plate glass windows on two sides, which offered a beautiful nighttime view of the city lights of Birmingham.

"Good evening, Mr. Burcham. It's good to see you again," Tracy said, as she helped the orderly guide the bed into position against the wall next to the monitoring equipment, electrical connections, examining lights, vacuum and oxygen ports. "I hear you are doing great on your first day post-transplant, and I'm going to be with you all night long."

After she got me hooked up to the monitoring systems, she took my vital signs and gave me my medications. And she kept her promise, literally. Wired on steroids, I was unable to sleep, and Tracy stayed up with me throughout her shift. When she wasn't performing her duties, we talked about my health, heart transplant patients in general and the recovery process, not to mention our families, careers, kids, significant others—we covered just about all the important matters in our lives.

In the morning, Doug replaced her as my nurse, along with Hart, a burly technician who popped into my brightly sunlit corner room with a smile and an armload of fresh towels and washing gear.

"Time for your bath, Mr. Burcham," he declared cheerfully.

I didn't know how I felt about getting washed by a male technician, but I needn't have worried. Before long Hart had a towel draped over my shoulders and was washing my hair with the warmest, soapiest water I'd ever experienced, and it felt wonderful. The shave was a little rough, though. It seems that we all develop a shaving routine that follows the natural contours of our faces comfortably, but when someone else is maneuvering the razor, it's not always smooth sailing; although it was worth enduring to get all the stubble off my face.

There was one area that went untouched for a while, however: The right side of my neck where a clear bandage covered the entryway of a huge port and manifold, dangling with tubes. Frankenstein, with a few zipper scars and a couple of pegs in his neck, had nothing on me!

Soon I was standing buck naked on towels spread on the floor, looking out the window down 6th Avenue while Hart washed me from head to toe. Nearly finished, he asked, "Do you want to wash the boys?" and I quickly took over and finished the process.

With his help, I put my flannel pajama bottoms back on with a fresh gown over them and went to sit in the chair for a while.

Doug brought me breakfast and my meds. We immediately hit it off. He was about my height, but a little stockier, wore glasses and a sunny disposition, and had the same situational sense of humor that I did. I found out that he liked good wine, nice restaurants and best of all, was an avid Auburn fan. We both had undergraduate degrees from the University of Alabama and master's degrees from Auburn University, which is rare down south—you're either Alabama or Auburn all the way.

In addition to his duties at UAB, Doug was a nursing professor at Jefferson State, a local community college. When I told him my undergraduate degree was in engineering, he began to give me lots of data about heart transplants and explained the "why" behind every aspect of my surgery and recovery.

So when he told me, "Steve, don't push yourself up with your arms right now," he followed up with the clinical reason why I shouldn't do so.

One time when he came into the room, he found me reclined in the chair attempting to pull myself up with both arms and hands, and he called out, "Steve, be careful! You are going to unleash a poltergeist!"

Hurrying over to help me get upright, he pointed at the eight-inch incision scar in my chest, visible through the drooping neckline of my hospital gown, and continued, "You have to be careful with that chest wound. It can spring a leak. I've seen patients trying to sit up on their own and all of a sudden, phiisst, phiisst!"—he made the sounds with the tip of his tongue visible between his clenched teeth—"blood will shoot straight across the room, just like a poltergeist!"

I burst out laughing, which hurt worse than coughing, which led to another, teary-eyed laughing fit. Doug handed me my "cough" pillow—a heart-shaped cushion that my neighbor, also named Doug, had brought for me—helped me settle down and just stood there looking at me with a knowing grin.

When you wake up from heart surgery, one of the first things you notice is that it hurts to inhale and exhale fully, cough, sneeze or laugh—in that order. Breathing is uncomfortable, sneezing and laughing are downright painful. I learned to keep my "cough" pillow handy when friends called me on the phone because they invariably told me a joke or story to try to cheer me up and make me laugh. If I detected that I might need to cough or sneeze, I'd grab the pillow and clamp it between my crossed arms and hands and squeeze it hard into my chest. That diminished the flexure of my chest and limited the level of pain—in theory. I found that for maximum comfort, I had to also bend over with my forearms braced in my lap. If the urge came on too sudden, I'd just cross my arms sans pillow and hope for the best.

As I settled into the routine, I learned that nurses and technicians worked 12-hour shifts, three days on, four days off. The schedule rotated from week to week.

On Thursday, Amber, a young blonde with a cute smile and a sparkle in her eyes, was my day nurse. She was a little more serious than Tracy and Doug. Sometimes she would think first before laughing at my jokes and barbs, making clear with an eye-roll or exasperated look what she really thought of them. She was something of a perfectionist with her relentless attention to detail, a strict adherence to the schedule, and the need to do things right every time. There were no short cuts or leeway when she was on the floor.

If I said, "Let's wait until tomorrow to change that PICC line dressing, it looks fine," Amber would respond, "It's been on for three days. It's time for a dressing change. Put up your computer, recline that bed back and get ready for me to change it right now, Mr. Burcham."

Still, I appreciated her, as I came to value every nurse and technician in the HTICU. Each one brought a different perspective and a wealth of experience to my situation. The collective body of knowledge that came into my room through these caregivers gave me as thorough a grounding as I needed to develop an actionable recovery plan for myself.

I was excited the morning Dr. Tallaj and Dr. Pamboukian did their rounds and, after examining me, turned to their entourage of residents and gave the order to "pull his tubes." I finally would have some mobility again! I could hardly wait for the nurse practitioner to unhook me so I could get up and move around the unit. Part of the recovery plan was to walk, walk, walk, and walk. The doctors wanted patients to be active and mobile. They wanted to see if my cardiovascular system was functioning well enough and make sure my legs hadn't gotten too weak. Walking was one of the keys to eventually being discharged.

Cindy and Yen were visiting when Elizabeth, the nurse practitioner, looking doctoral in her white lab coat, entered the room, and said, "Mr. Burcham it's time to get those tubes out. Are you ready?"

"You bet. Where are we going to do the procedure?"

"Right here. Put away your stuff and recline flat in your bed. We have to create a sterile zone over here."

As I stretched out on the bed with only my pajama bottoms on, tubes and wires exposed, Yen and Elizabeth donned masks, hairnets and surgical gowns. They approached me with towels and cleaning swabs while Amber stood at the supply cabinet behind them, ready to replenish as needed. Elizabeth spread a thick layer of towels just below my sternum where the two main tubes—each about the diameter of a pinky finger—were protruding from my chest. Then she grabbed the tube on the left, looked up, said "Here goes," and pulled until it was completely out.

Immediately, she began to apply pressure with a pile of gauze about a half-inch thick to the opening in my skin, sopping up any remaining fluid. After about 10 minutes of keeping pressure on, she looked down and said, "Nice."

She grasped the tube on the right and gave it a steady tug, pulling it slowly out of position. I heard a gushing sound like a brief burst of running water, and the words you never want to hear in a hospital, "Gee, I've never seen *that* before."

Yen replied, "Well, you *have* to pull it the rest of the way out."

What emerged from the hole in my lower right chest looked like a thick, red spaghetti noodle.

Meanwhile Yen provided commentary for Cindy and me, "Eew, Mr. Burcham, you just delivered a 'goo' baby!"

"That's weird," Elizabeth reported as she lowered the stringy object onto the towel.

"Can I take a look?" I asked.

"Sure, if you can stomach it," Yen replied as Elizabeth and Amber went about applying pressure, and swabbing and dressing the two openings in my chest.

As I peered over them working, I saw something that looked like a blood-red, thin, long sock with fluid bulging and dripping from the bottom.

Elizabeth explained that this was the result of blood that had coagulated like a sock around the tube inside me. When she pulled on the tube, the "sock" came off leaving the top visible outside of my body. When she pulled the sock out, I delivered a "goo baby."

"It's a good thing Mrs. Burcham delivered your daughters, because they sure would be ugly if you had done the job!" Yen commented with a smile.

After the excitement of the delivery wore off, Elizabeth gave me the not-so-good news. "Mr. Burcham, I know you are ready to start walking, but based on what just happened, I need you to lie flat. We'll restart quarter-hour vital checks for the rest of first shift, just to be on the safe side, OK?" she said sternly.

Having to wait once more was agony, but by early evening, I was finally cleared for my first "outing." Chris, the male nurse on call, delivered my medications and said, "Mr. Burcham, I've heard you are ready to start walking. I'll get my other patient taken care of and come back in a little while with a walker so we can get you up and around the unit."

"Don't bother bringing that thing. I won't need a walker," I snapped.

"Yes, sir. It will have to be arm-in-arm then with you, you know."

"Yes, but no walker."

The house lights were off in the unit—bedtime—when Chris returned around 10:30 p.m. "Are you ready to do a few laps, Mr. Burcham?"

"You bet! I really wanted to get started today so I can build upon my progress tomorrow and over the weekend," I said excitedly.

Moving my intravenous medication pole over to the right side of the bed, Chris put his strong arm around my back to get me the rest of the way out of the bed and into a standing position. After a few brief adjustments, we took the first steps, arm in arm, to the inside door of the airlock entryway. By now, all visitors had departed, and the only folks who saw my inaugural walk with a new heart were Chris and the other nurses working the unit.

As I made it out through the second door of the airlock, we met Roman, another nurse. He smiled and said, "Way to go, Mr. Burcham, we knew it wouldn't be any time at all before you would be up and getting around! Go for it!"

The HTICU was comprised of a dozen or so patient rooms arranged along a U-shaped hallway with nurses' stations and offices, and a coffee klatch employee break area in the center. The hallway had two crossways which intersected the U once near the entrance and again about halfway up the sides. A "lap" consisted of walking the biggest possible loop of the U without leaving the unit. Twenty laps added up to one mile. With Chris' help, I managed to make it slowly around once. My legs felt like I was carrying a gallon of milk tied to each one, but my heart felt fine. I was thoroughly satisfied with my performance as I settled back into bed. "Tomorrow, I'll shoot for ten laps or one-half a mile," I thought as I started to flip through the channels on television.

I didn't meet my goal the next day, but I was up to a mile and a half, a half mile more than the doctors' challenge, in no time.

I was surprised how free of heart symptoms I was during the first week post-transplant. Except for some minor body aches, I experienced no pain and was making steady progress physically. At the same time, I didn't expect the flood of emotions that would come on suddenly without warning, and bring me to tears.

One time I was sitting on the edge of my bed, head down, trying to finish my lunch with tears dripping down onto the paper-lined cafeteria tray, when Lindsey entered the room.

"Why is Dad crying?" she asked.

Sniffling, I tried to pull myself together. "I don't know why I'm crying! Who cries while they are eating ice cream? And they gave me *two* cardboard cups of vanilla today, not just one."

As she made her way to the chair across the room, Cindy half-whispered to her "It started a few minutes ago right before you entered. He said he didn't have a sad thought in his head, nothing to be unhappy about, yet when he got to his dessert, he just broke down in tears. I believe it's all the steroids he's taking every day for rejection. He's been very emotional this week."

Lindsey grinned and called to me, "Hey, Dad, now you know how all of us girls feel—hormones generating emotions from nowhere!"

But it was more than that. While the medications could have been a convenient excuse for a guy "who wasn't supposed to cry," I realized quickly that I was shedding both tears of joy and sadness for the donor and his family, who despite their suffering and grief, had lovingly bestowed a miraculous gift on an unknown recipient.

One of the doctors, who liked to be called by his first name, Deepak, and I had many conversations about treatment, meds, side effects and human physiology.

Early one morning I was doing my laps, and he was working at one of the computer consoles. When I said hello, he asked if I had any questions. Needless to say, I fired off a bevy. As he pulled up my records, he volunteered without prompting, "Your donor was 22 years old and had the same blood type. Everything matched perfectly." That's how I found out my donor's age.

Deepak continued, "Also, the donor had been exposed to CMV. Since you haven't, that could present a small hurdle in the future."

He explained that CMV—cytomegalovirus—is a common virus that many of us are exposed to when we are young. I was one of a small segment of the population who hadn't been exposed, so my new heart might give me CMV in the future. I was taking Valcyte, a powerful antiviral medicine that prevents it, but the risk of contracting it would increase when the doctors took me off it after my one-year heart transplant anniversary.

I decided that was one of the bridges to cross when I came to it. In the meantime, I started to reflect on my donor, whose life had ended so that mine could continue, and every time I talked to someone about it, tears would well up.

The following Monday, Doug brought his six nursing students for a visit. They had donned white gowns with their names on right breast pockets and "Jefferson State University" boldly displayed on the left side. Doug was particularly interested in having them interview a heart transplant patient who was progressing well just six days after surgery and who could explain the post-operative treatment plan with detail about the various medications that are prescribed and their purposes.

From my bed I briefly recounted my health journey, allowing everyone to ask questions along the way. Then I continued with a tearful account of "how I had felt" the days after receiving a new donor heart. Drying my eyes with a tissue, I composed myself and got down to the technical aspects of the cocktail of drugs I was on.

Picking up my pill bottles one at a time, I first explained about CellCept, Prograf and prednisone, which I was taking to prevent organ rejection. Then I pointed to another set of medicines and continued, "Since the first three drugs suppress my immune system, this group here are my antifungal, antibacterial, antiviral and anti-yeast drugs."

Finally, I directed their attention to my bedside table, concluding, "The balance of bottles over here are dietary supplements and antacids for my digestive system."

After the students asked a few follow-up questions, they commented on how well I looked and how well I was doing, and wished me luck. Doug thanked me with a wink as he trailed the group back through the airlock and into the hallway.

Alone again, I mused about the remarkable developments in medicine and pharmaceuticals that had given me a new lease on life. At the same time, it was crystal clear to me that God's unconditional, unbounded love was the only reason all of this had happened successfully. I realized I wasn't out of the woods yet, but I trusted that through His grace and peace, I would remain unrattled and confident during the good and bad times ahead. I knew He was in control and would be there for me every step of the way.

CHAPTER 11

"NEW NORMAL" IN BIRMINGHAM

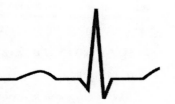

On the morning of Tuesday, February 21, bright winter sunshine streamed into the Presidential Suite. Cindy was reading her Kindle as she sat curled up in the chair opposite from me, cell phone charging in her lap. I lounged fully dressed in another chair, feet propped up on the hospital bed, while I pecked away at my laptop keyboard in regard to various issues at Digium that needed tending to.

On Sunday I had walked 60 laps around the unit—the equivalent of three miles—setting a record. The doctors told me not to go for 80 laps because if news got out, it might upset the other patients. I offered to donate the extras to a "lap bank" that the others could use as needed to reach their goals, but the doctors didn't warm up to the idea.

At some point, Dr. Pamboukian entered the room, her entourage of nurses, interns and residents in tow.

"Working again?" she inquired.

"Yep, just catching up on e-mail." Following up with my usual banter, I added, "Dr. Pamboukian, why don't you let me out of here and give this room to someone who is *really* sick and needs it?"

She nodded and a smile flitted across her normally serious face. "Mr. Burcham, you are going to get your wish. You are doing well. Yesterday, your rejection level was 1R, indicating that a mild level of rejection is present, but that's not unexpected. We will measure it again next Monday, then every Monday for the next five weeks and take action if necessary. So, let me examine you real quick."

Watching me struggle out of my clothes, she commented, "That is why we like our patients in their gowns."

While she checked on my heart, she continued to explain. "We'll get you out of here by noon, which is only six and a half days post-operation—quite impressive. By the way, we are going to count this week as your first week 'in clinic,' so you and Cindy will need to stay in the Birmingham area for this week plus five more. You'll be visiting us two or three days per week. Dana will review your complete schedule with you before you leave today."

Finishing up, she wrapped her stethoscope around her neck. "Any questions?"

"Can I have a cold beer when I leave?" I said with a grin.

"Drink O'Doul's. You know, you're in the Presidential Suite, and President Bush drank O'Doul's; you should learn to like it, too."

"O'Doul's tastes like seltzer water," I protested.

"Then drink seltzer water."

"OK, I got the message. No cold beer."

"Not until you get out of clinic. Wait five weeks. We are hammering your kidneys and liver right now with these medications. We can talk again before you leave Birmingham."

I nodded in agreement as she and her staff left. Then the reality of what she'd said earlier sunk in: I was going to leave the hospital a new man and start the journey to return to my normal life!

Of course, nothing happens quickly in a hospital unless there is a crisis. Amber refused to pull my PICC, the only set of tubes still dangling from my body, until she saw the doctor's signature on the discharge papers. Once they arrived, she went into action like clockwork.

Then Dana stopped by for a half-hour education session. She covered everything from medications, to dos and don'ts, to important phone numbers, to clinic appointments and how to prepare for them. It was the longest 30 minutes of my stay, and by the end my head was pounding.

At the end, a witness and I had to sign off that I had received her set of instructions. "I just need to get away from all of this for a while!" I screamed internally as I scribbled my signature at the bottom of the sheet.

By now it was early afternoon, and all my belongings had been loaded on a pushcart. I was ready to bolt, but there was one final requirement, as Amber informed me.

"You have to ring the bell. It's tradition," she insisted. "We'll call all the available caregivers in the HTICU over to the counter, and then you ring the big brass bell to announce that you are leaving. In return, we'll provide parting applause and hugs!"

After everyone gathered around the bell, Cindy snapped a photo when I pulled the cord. Immediately afterward, I took off my surgical mask—I wanted everyone to see me smiling ear to ear. The applause was joyful and heartfelt (pun intended).

As we exited the unit, I texted the photo Cindy had taken of me at the bell to a dozen close friends and family members with a short note that I was being discharged. At six and a half days, I now held the record for the shortest stay in the HTICU after a heart transplant at UAB.

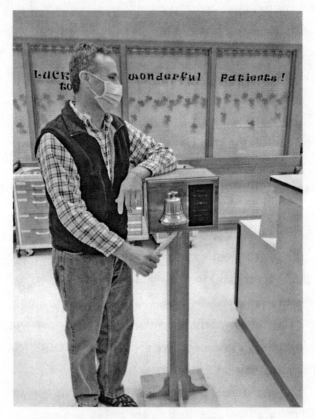

Ringing the "freedom bell"

The weather outside was crisp and unseasonably warm. Amber kept me company while we waited for Cindy to bring the car around from the parking garage. I could tell she was enjoying the little break from work on the unit. By then I was wearing my mask again, and we made small talk until our SUV rounded the corner. Amber gave me a quick hug and wished me good luck. With her help I climbed into the car, and Cindy and I were on our way.

As we drove toward the Bell Summit apartment complex, where we'd be spending the next five weeks, Cindy asked what we should do about lunch. I could tell she was a bit surprised when I suggested Wendy's.

"That's right, I want a Wendy's number one combo meal with cheese, French fries and a sweet tea," I insisted.

"OK, I know you haven't had a treat like that in over six months, so I'll go through the drive-thru and we'll take our lunch to our apartment and eat it there."

After picking up the food, we got off the main highway and drove through Cahaba Heights to our new home away from home. Along the way, I started to feel nauseous.

"Cindy, I *never* get carsick, but today your driving is killing me! Can you just slow down around all these curves and hills?"

"Wow, that's a first; my driving making you sick."

By the time we got to the ground-level, one-bedroom apartment, I was feeling better. We sat outside on the tiny back porch and dug into our lunch sacks. I was in for another unpleasant surprise. Everything tasted burnt—the burger, cheese and fries.

"And for the last week, I thought it was that darn hospital food!" I complained.

"Wait a minute, I'll be right back," Cindy said and went inside. She soon returned with a Kit Kat bar, a Milky Way and a scoop of vanilla ice cream.

"See how these taste," she said, handing me the Kit Kat bar.

I took one bite.

"Burnt and metallic."

The Milky Way and the ice cream tasted the same.

"How can ice cream taste like it's burned?"

"It has to be the medicines," Cindy declared.

I only managed to finish half of my lunch before I crumpled up the whole bag in frustration and tossed it into the trash can.

Fortunately, Ellen Martin, Digium's HR benefits manager, arrived just at the right time to take my mind off the disappointment. She and Timo Sandritter, the HR director, had put together a company-wide donation drive to support our six-week stay in Birmingham. The apartment was fully furnished but lacked everyday amenities like paper products, detergents, bottled water, utensils and cookware. Ellen was acting as the Good Samaritan, bringing us a supply of what we needed along with spices, frozen meats, canned goods and snacks. We simply had a wonderful bunch of friends at Digium!

"Great," I said. "Let's help her unload."

"You're not unloading anything," Cindy said. "Remember, you cannot lift anything heaver than a gallon of milk right now: doctor's orders."

Not lifting or pulling had headed the list of dos and don'ts Dana had gone over with us before my discharge. Some of the items were the same for anyone who had undergone open heart surgery with his rib cage cracked open—no lifting, opening twist-top jars or turning door knobs.

Others were specific to heart transplant patients. They included wearing a surgical mask outdoors and in public and keeping my hands sanitized. I wasn't to shake hands with anyone, and if I forgot, I must wash or wipe them down right away. If my eyes itched, I was to use my sleeve or a Kleenex to rub them rather than my fingers.

I'd been told to avoid superstores like Walmart and church services. Apparently, they are hotbeds of bacteria and viruses because people go to both even when they are sick.

When dining out, we were to go during non-peak hours and *never* to buffet-type establishments. During our time in Birmingham, we usually had dinner at 4 p.m. I'd wear my mask into the restaurant and would take it off after sitting down.

Certain fare was off-limits *now and forever*. Any item from a salad bar, raw or undercooked food like sushi and rare steak, raw fruit unless it had been thoroughly washed, leftovers that had sat for more than a day or two, and grapefruit, which produced a negative reaction with one of my medications.

I wasn't to clean toilets or have cats and litter boxes in the house ever again. If I wanted to go swimming, it was in pools and oceans only, never in lakes, rivers, streams, ponds or other stagnant waters. Going on cruise ship vacations was a no-no forever, too.

One item was Steve Burcham-specific. I couldn't scuba dive anymore. Dana told me that a young female heart transplant patient lost her life after getting sick from the equipment and compressed air. Although I understood that it was just too risky, having to give up one of my favorite pastimes saddened me greatly.

There were other dos and don'ts I learned to observe along the way, but the primary lessons were that hand cleanliness was the real key to avoiding sickness, and that a little paranoia goes a long way. I believe that the surgical mask was more about warning others to stay away, though, to create a do-not-cross boundary; and it worked like a charm: Folks in public would not even make eye contact with me when I was wearing my face protector.

As we settled into a daily routine, Cindy and I quickly realized that the small four-chair dinette set in the apartment wasn't big enough to serve as my desk, her desk and our occasional eating area. In addition, we had conflicting telephone styles. Cindy was matter-of-fact, but liked to turn up the volume. I tended to get passionate and paced a lot. To help us achieve some physical separation, her mom brought me a card table from home, which I set up in the opposite corner of the main room next to the small entertainment center and the exit to the patio. That way, if I needed to pace while on my cell phone, I could take it outside.

Charlie Wilson, Digium's hardware engineering manager, sent me the company's latest technology, a mid-line business telephone pre-programmed with my work extension. He had won the "Guess When Steve is Going to Get a New Heart" contest that was started at the company just days before I got the donor call. By then only two employees had time to submit their dates: Charlie and Barbara Duffey, Digium's controller. Her guess was February 14, which was the day I woke up from the operation; but technically I received the new heart on the 13th, so Charlie was declared the winner.

With my new Digium D50 telephone and laptop computer, I was ready to get back into the thick of things, so I typed out an e-mail to Danny and Timo:

Now that Cindy and I are settled into our apartment here in Birmingham, I would like to propose the following back-to-work plan and schedule. For the rest of February and all of March, I will be "in clinic" on Mondays and Thursdays and will be unavailable for work on those days. However, on Tuesdays, Wednesdays and Fridays, I will be available and would like to work remotely. My desk telephone is now operational here in Birmingham. My schedule is up-to-date

with my appointments, proposed days off, and days available.
I plan to return to work full time and be back in my office at
headquarters on April 2, 2012.

> *Thank you,*
> *Steve*

Danny's quick response expressed both concern and support. He worried that I was pushing myself a bit too hard, but deferred to my judgment. If this was the pace of recovery I wanted, he would back me up. He also made the point that if I needed to slow down at anytime, I should feel free to do so.

During my time in the apartment in Birmingham, I had 19 full-day visits to the five-story Kirklin Clinic at UAB, a self-contained mini medical mall with several departments on each floor. On 12 of those visits, I underwent right heart catheterizations (RHC), during which the doctors inserted a catheter into the right side of my neck, accessed the interior of my heart through a vein, and used tiny forceps on the tip to remove four small pieces of tissue from the donor heart. These samples were then sent to pathology and examined microscopically for early signs of rejection. The scale is as follows: 0R = no rejection, 1R = slight rejection, 2R = moderate rejection, 3R = severe rejection. My reading of 1R at my first RHC on the Monday before my discharge was of no concern—apparently, 95% of patients experience some level of rejection during the first year post-operation. Only levels 2R or 3R merit treatment.

On clinic days, I usually got up before dawn, showered and made coffee. Then I woke up Cindy as I barged through the bedroom door from the hallway bath to our apartment's master bedroom to get dressed. By 6:30 a.m. we were on our way making the 12-minute trip downtown to Kirklin Clinic. During rush hour or at lunchtime it would easily have been a 30-minute drive.

Mondays were always a full day in clinic for me. My schedule included visits to five departments on three floors. The blood analysis laboratory was always stop number one. Since it was almost right inside the front entrance, it was impossible to forget to have one's "labs drawn." After the labs, I was scheduled to go to the third floor for a chest X-ray, then one floor up to cardiovascular and pulmonary for an RHC, echo and EKG; then over to the pharmacist's office for a quick review of my medications, and finally to an examining room on the top floor for a quick visit with my transplant coordinator and cardiologist.

On our first visit, we arrived early and were the last to leave. Based on that experience, we figured there must be a "secret" to navigating the maze of tests and appointments. It wasn't long before we caught on—if you were not first or second in line, it would be a long day for you. The strategy we learned was to go sign in everywhere, a task Cindy graciously decided to do for me. Since the computer system knew where I was in the lineup of tests, the nurses in each department didn't strike my name off the list. They simply called for me again later on if I didn't put in an appearance on the first round. The quickest we were able to make it through the labyrinthine course and get out of clinic was four hours; the longest time it took was seven hours.

As we walked in from the parking deck, Cindy headed for the centrally located elevators to sign the registers on the third and fourth floors, while I went directly to get my labs drawn. We agreed to meet on the fourth floor.

The blood analysis lab and X-ray were the fastest departments. The bottleneck usually occurred with the right heart catheterization (RHC), which was done in the operating room. Sometimes they had a half dozen of us heart transplant patients stacked up for the procedure, so if you weren't first or second in line, you could count on spending the rest of the day catching up.

We made good time that day. After all labs, tests and procedures were completed, we went to see the doctor to make sure everything was progressing well. As Cindy and I waited in the examining room, we heard some shuffling feet in the hallway, followed by a quick knock, and Dr. Pamboukian entered trailed by Dr. Le, who made his way to the counter, sat down and began logging on to the computer.

Dr. Pamboukian placed her stethoscope under the back of my shirt and instructed me to take slow breaths in and out to listen to my lungs.

"Good, your lungs sound clear," she said.

At her direction, I lay down to have her squeeze my ankles to feel for fluid buildup and then to listen to my heart and stomach. Then she had me turn my head to check the veins in my neck.

"You can sit up, Mr. Burcham," she concluded. "You look great. How do you feel?"

"Just as you say!" I said.

I caught her up on my walking up to two miles per day without any cardiac symptoms like shortness of breath or dizziness. The only medication side effects I was experiencing were a little shakiness in my hands and the dulling of my taste buds. I mentioned that my legs still felt weak and that I had a tender area on the back of my left leg calf, probably from walking too much; and finished up that my blood pressure was running on the high side of normal.

By then, Dr. Le had finished at the computer and joined Dr. Pamboukian by my exam table. "Steve, all your bloodwork, heart tests, X-rays—perfect! You are going to live a long, long time with your heart!" he said, grinning from ear to ear.

Dr. Pamboukian recapped cautiously, in counterpoint to his upbeat tone, "Dr. Le and Dana have checked all your tests and everything looks fine. Your rejection level has now dropped to 0R, and all your organ functions look fine. We'll just continue to monitor your blood pressure and treat it if it rises or doesn't settle into the normal range soon. Remember, things can change fast, so simply live your life and don't worry. If anything happens, we'll be here to help."

When she finished with her usual, "Any questions for me?" I was ready. "When can I start jogging?" I asked.

"You need to wait 12 weeks post-operation before you start jogging or swinging a golf club, no exceptions," she said sternly. "Besides, being low on magnesium, you'll likely experience some cramping in your muscles."

"Do you think I will be able to *run* a five-kilometer race on Memorial Day?"

"Well, you've demonstrated the ability to *walk* more than two kilometers in ICU just five days post-op, so I think you'll be fine on Memorial Day. We'll continue to monitor your progress and let's agree to talk about it before you go home," she concluded.

I was putting on a good face in a frustrating situation. My legs were still very weak and often felt numb, which surprised me considering I had been off them for only three days following surgery. I wondered what happened to patients who were bedridden for weeks or months! At first, when I started walking outside at the apartment at what seemed like a snail's pace, Cindy had to come along and hold my hand. It took a week before I was able to go out on my own and not have to halt every 100 yards or so to rest. It took even longer before I managed half a mile without stopping. Eventually I worked myself up to two miles a day.

In addition to numbness in my legs, I often experienced tingling and random cramps all over my body. Sometimes the tingling would start in my feet and travel all the way to my cranium before subsiding. I felt cramps in my limbs, chest and back muscles, but they were most pronounced in my fingers and toes; they would come on suddenly and often, and go away just as quickly. My taste buds were returning to normal, albeit very slowy. I was wired and hungry all the time. Trips to the DQ for a chocolate milkshake to satisfy my intense craving became an afternoon ritual!

I became moody and emotional without apparent reason. Sometimes, I got frustrated at Cindy about nothing and would snap at her, only to ask her forgiveness moments later. At night, I managed no more than five hours of sleep, and for the first time in my life, had very detailed dreams, some in color, some black and white.

One particularly vivid dream remains as crystal clear in my mind now as it was the day I awakened from restless sleep in our apartment about a week or two after surgery. It was a scene like out of the movie "Inception," but in black and white. I found myself sitting in a sparsely furnished doctor's office. There were chairs along the walls and in the middle of the room, a door to the doctor's examining areas, and an opaque, grayish white receptionist window. No one was behind the glass. A young person, about my height and build, with long, dark brown hair, was next to me. We did not talk or look at one another, but simply sat quietly and stared straight ahead, waiting together until I got called. The scene cross-faded and I was suddenly looking out from inside my open chest cavity. I could see two shadows on either side of me, peering into my chest—they were surgeons. One worked for a while, and then paused. Then the other took over while the first surgeon assisted. This went on for some time before I woke up feeling calm and contemplative.

I have often wondered about this dream since and pondered its meaning from time to time. I believe the young person was my heart donor, but beyond that, I have not been able to make sense of it.

Meanwhile, the visits to the Kirklin Clinic continued like clockwork, even on my birthday. I knew I was going to have a fun time when I walked into the heart catheter lab and Dr. Cadeiras had birthday music playing on the loudspeakers in the operating room.

"Y'all remembered!"

"It's not that hard, Mr. Burcham. Your date of birth is all over the computer screens and charts," Dr. Cadeiras said, smiling, as I removed my shirt and prepared to lie down on the operating room table for my weekly RHC and biopsy.

"You guys don't even give us heart transplant patients a break on our birthdays, do you?" I mock complained.

Dr. Cadeiras misunderstood my tone of voice. "Mr. Burcham," he said seriously. "You should be happy you are here on your birthday. Remember what shape you were in back in November, just four months ago today?"

"You're right! I have a lot to be thankful for—I can't think of anywhere else I would rather be," I said dryly.

Once again, my procedure, labs, tests and doctor's visit proved normal, and Cindy and I returned to our apartment, where the long string of planned "birthday surprises" that had been hatched without my knowledge, began.

First, we were greeted by an overnight package on the doorstep. Inside, I found a supersized, handmade birthday card signed by the employees at Digium and a CD.

Cindy read the comments out loud while I popped the CD in my laptop to watch the video.

It was a montage of employees from both Digium's San Diego and Huntsville locations wishing me "Happy Birthday" to soft background music. The HR department must have put an inordinate amount of time into capturing so many well wishers. It was priceless and very moving.

My favorite was, "Your body is fifty; your new heart is half that age. You have the mindset of a fourteen-year-old, so your average age is twenty-one. Enjoy your birthday!"

"That guy knows you too well, doesn't he?" Cindy said, laughing.

About the time the video finished, Brooke knocked on the door for a surprise visit. We replayed the video for her and then went out for a birthday lunch together.

Later there were more surprises. Anna and Jake arrived from Auburn, and Cindy presented me with more than 90 birthday cards she had been collecting in secret over the last week. I had wondered why she didn't want me to pick up the mail on my walks; now I knew. One day, she actually had left a few cards in the mailbox and let me pick them up so I wouldn't get suspicious or think everyone had forgotten my birthday.

Then, as I spent the next hour or so going through all the cards, our good friends Buddy and Carole arrived with gifts and an invitation to dinner. I managed to talk everyone into going to my favorite Italian restaurant so that I could get my favorite dish: penne pasta with shrimp, chicken, prosciutto, cheese and Alfredo sauce. Cindy let me have my first glass of red wine since the surgery.

Back at the apartment, I opened all of my gifts and declared, "This has been the best birthday ever!"

It was also a welcome break in what had become an intense regimen for me. I had to take 12 medications three times a day *unfailingly*. Even missing just one could propel me into a state of rejection. I quickly realized that the maintenance on my new heart would require a fundamentally different approach than I was used to. This was unlike taking care of my car or home, where I might sometimes let the "change oil" light stay on too long, or allow the paint to weather, peel and flake. Perhaps aircraft maintenance, in which systems and components were checked and overhauled on an "hours of usage" basis, was a model on par with transplant organ maintenance. It was a daunting task.

Fortunately, I had some idea that in time, things would get easier. At clinic one day, I met a guy about my age who was nine years out with his new heart. His morning medication regimen consisted of three pills only. He also pointed out that visits to the clinic became annual, and the number of medications required had gone down to those of a typical heart patient— encouraging indeed.

All of this talk about heart maintenance got me thinking, "What does maintaining our faith look like?" I didn't think I'd find the word in the index of my Bible or concordance. "Maintenance" as in "sustaining," yes; but "maintenance" as in "working at it daily," not so much—something to keep pondering.

At some point, I realized that my health crisis was actually a blessing on another front. It has allowed me to address my concern of our transition from full-time parents back to a full-time couple in a positive way. Six months earlier I had wondered what we were going to do with ourselves after the kids moved along into adulthood. After 27 years of marriage, would we try to rediscover each other in a new way? Could we rekindle the magic that had drawn us together in the jewelry store where we had worked and met as teenagers?

The good news was that Cindy and I were spending more time alone together than we ever had in the past, even before we had our girls. The only sad part—it was in Birmingham rather than the Bahamas! We went to movies, found new restaurants, planned to buy board games we used to enjoy before the kids, like Trivial Pursuit, and researched places for a summer family vacation.

One weekend, we just drove around the neighborhoods of Birmingham, sightseeing. Another, we took advantage of the unseasonably warm weather and visited the botanical gardens to look at the azaleas. As we walked toward the entrance of the gardens, the gift shop caught Cindy's eye and we took a brief detour. When we spotted a Bloodgood Japanese Maple tree ready to plant, we agreed that there was a perfect spot for it in Madison in the flower bed outside my study window and vowed to pick it up on our way home later in the month.

There were times when I simply marveled at Cindy's determination and commitment. Except for a few hours to travel home or to go to the store, she did not leave my side unless someone else was with me. She supported me then and has always provided balance and foundation to my more mercurial approach to life.

While being a husband and father has always been a priority to me, in practice, for many years of our lives together, Cindy focused on the kids and I, somewhat selfishly, focused on my career. Anna was born with a heart murmur that needed to be monitored. When she was a toddler and had to be taken to the hospital with a high fever, it was Cindy who did that while I was heading to the airport to catch a plane to Detroit for an important "business meeting and golf outing."

When Cindy recently reminded me of that occasion, I was thankful that she added, "You are not the same person—you wouldn't do that today."

Hmm, give up golf? Not sure.

If I have to be honest, I must admit that I was no paragon of virtue, and Cindy was not superwoman. We were just two tenacious high school sweethearts who, with the help of family, friends and the Lord, had come a long way together, and hopefully had a long way to go.

Perhaps there was some greater purpose at work when I received my new heart just before Valentine's Day; I vowed that from now on I'd show my life partner how much she meant to me as often as possible.

Toward the end of our stay in Birmingham in late March, Cindy surprised me. When I asked if she were ready to take me to my regular cardiac physical therapy, she tossed me the car keys and said, "I think I'll stay here and catch up on doing our bills."

"Wow," I thought. "I can't believe this. My primary caregiver is letting me out on the town by myself. I should hit the Irish pub in the Summit for a few hours and come back a little tipsy, just to see the reaction on her face!"

Climbing behind the wheel of Cindy's SUV wasn't the same as sitting in my Jeep, but driving by myself gave me a feeling of normalcy and freedom I hadn't experienced in a long time. I opened the sunroof to enjoy the warm spring weather, cranked up some XM on Cindy's Bose stereo and just enjoyed the drive. By the time I got to the Spain Rehabilitation Center, I was flying high.

Christie, one of the trainers, welcomed me, "Hello, Mr. Burcham. Jason generated your exercise plan for the next 15 weeks. If you are up to it, we are going to push you a bit today!"

"Bring it on!" I said.

Christie was in her mid-20s, a bubbly, tall, athletic blonde, who turned bright red at the slightest kidding or joking. Needless to say, I took every opportunity I could to tease her and make her blush.

After putting on my heart monitor and having her check my vitals, I got started on the treadmill. There were three other patients waiting next to me who were easily 10 years older than me—familiar faces from previous workouts. One, a thin, tall woman, was being qualified for a heart transplant. Another was a petite woman who had decided against a lung transplant seven years earlier and had exceeded everyone's expectations by continuing to live. The third was a short, burly county sheriff who always showed up in full uniform before changing into his workout clothes.

"OK, Christie," I teased, loud enough for everyone to hear. "Just tell the sheriff he won't have to hold a gun to my back; I'll promise to get my heart rate into the desirable range. You know he's packing heat today!"

"That's right, Christie," the sheriff called out as he pushed forward on the exercise machine.

"Yeah, and my wife let me out on my own today," I continued. "I thought about blowing today's session off and heading to the pub for some beer, but I was afraid y'all would come looking for me and rat me out to Cindy!"

The exchange wasn't all that funny, but I noted with satisfaction that Christie was smiling and her face beet-red. Mission accomplished!

For the first five minutes, I worked my way from a casual to a brisk walk. Then I started ramping up the pace and the incline on the machine. Five minutes later, I called for my next vitals check.

"Push a little harder, Mr. Burcham, you are on the low end of your target range," Christie called out, not looking up from her workstation and monitor.

I pushed the incline to level five and the pace to four—a 13-minute mile—about as fast as I could go without breaking into a jog.

As I began to work up an actual cardiovascular sweat, Christie took my blood pressure, "One thirty-six over seventy-five, heart rate one-fifty-five—very good Mr. Burcham," she reported. "Finish your thirty minutes, cool down and we'll get you started on leg presses."

"Whew, she doesn't play around," I said to the miracle lung lady, who was on the treadmill next to me, oxygen lines in her nostrils, doing a one-hour workout.

I figured it was sheer tenacity that continued to extend her life. Her lung problems were self-induced: A heavy smoker and overweight, she opted not to take donor lungs away from other deserving patients. Instead, she quit cigarettes, lost 100 pounds, and was now happy as a lark, defying the odds every day. While she was doing fairly well, I'd seen half a dozen others in clinic wheezing and gasping for every breath.

I finished up my exercise routine for the day and said a final farewell to the team, "Folks, you know I've enjoyed getting to know all of you, but I'm being released later this week! Sorry I won't be able to hang in rehab with you anymore. My home gym won't be the same without you. Sheriff, keep your bullets in your pocket and Miss Smith, keep amazing everyone around you!"

And for Christie, a parting comment to make her blush: "I'm going to miss this personal attention you've been giving me; but it's better this way. My wife has been wondering why I come back so upbeat after my exercise sessions!"

On March 29, Dr. Pamboukian finally gave me the green light. I was free to leave Birmingham. Before Cindy and I left the medical campus, we dropped off a thank you card and some goodies for our friends in the HTICU.

As we were packing up the SUV for the trip home two days ahead of schedule, I sneaked back inside to update our friends and family via CaringBridge:

Through all of your e-mails, text messages, telephone calls, cards and guestbook posts, I have received many suggestions of what I should do next. Here is the list as I remember it:

- *Continue posting weekly on CaringBridge*

- *Start a personal spiritual-based blog*
- *Start teaching*
- *Start preaching*
- *Write a book*

I want to assure you that I have heard you and am prayerfully considering all of my options. I will comment on the first item, though—continue posting on CaringBridge—and let you know why I'm not going to do this.

The website was set up to help folks through a crisis of some sort—health, relationship, military deployment, etc. Hopefully, there is a defined beginning and ending; like "take cover" warnings we follow during inclement weather, at some point, we sound the "all clear." This allows us to be properly protected during dangerous times and then resume normal activities afterward. The way I see it, posting endlessly on CaringBridge is tantamount to declaring no end to the crisis. But even if my crisis hasn't completely subsided, I would like for my family and me to be able to resume a normal life anyway. As I've mentioned before, I'm so thankful that Danny set up the website for me, and that all of you built a protective "hedge of thorns" around us and prayed for us throughout this miraculous journey. We're grateful beyond measure!

So with this post I'm declaring "all clear!" I've resumed a new normal life and am going back to work!

Chapter 12
Wonderful Life Ahead

And that is exactly what I did. As planned, I returned to Digium on April 2, 2012, resumed my board positions at the Hogan YMCA in Madison and the Metro YMCA in Huntsville, and as Finance Committee Chairman of Asbury. There were plenty of challenges to keep me busy. Digium's business was soaring. Telephone manufacturing was behind, creating an order backlog that resulted in the need for additional capacity in China. The Metro YMCA was growing so fast, its chairman called several special planning sessions to sort out how we were going to manage the growth, keeping in mind the constraints every non-profit organization has to deal with.

On the family front, Lindsey and Jay started looking for their first house in Houston while Anna attended a summer program at Baylor, also in Houston, and Brooke was living back at home after graduating from Auburn searching for her first job. Cindy and I were deeply involved in all these activities. My calendar for the remainder of the year had very little white space on it.

The doctors had recommended that I stay away from Asbury until after Easter for two reasons. As I mentioned before, people aren't necessarily careful about going to church sick. More importantly, on my first day back, everyone would want to hug me and shake my hand. So we agreed to wait until the reports of my return to Madison had made the rounds and become old news, and aimed for a first visit in late April. But when Dad and Sara invited us to their church's outdoor Easter sunrise service, Cindy and I thought the health risk of me attending would be low, and we agreed to join them.

My dad spotted us arriving at the top of the hill and waved for us to join the family front and center about one third of the way down in the middle section of the amphitheater, which had been there as long as I can remember. Triangularly shaped and perched on the side of a mountain, it had a dramatic view of the valley below. The edges were of dry-stack rock, and the seats and stage backdrop were made of weatherworn concrete cinderblocks covered by a slight patchwork of moss. Dropping our blankets on the block seats in front of Dad and Sara, we had just enough room to squeeze in together.

After a few Easter hymns, a younger, hipper-looking man performed a guitar solo of "Watch the Lamb." It was the first time I ever heard the song and it resonated with me. At some point, the sun peeked over the tree line and began shedding light on the congregation. Reverend Dale Clem did a wonderful job of recounting Mary Magdalene's discovery of the empty tomb. During the sermon, he and I locked eyes for a moment. I knew I would get a chance to greet him after the service. Other than the reverend and my family, I only recognized two other Madison residents. "Three hugs after the service," I thought. "I'll be fine!"

Afterward we all piled back into our cars and traveled to my childhood home where Sara had arranged a small homecoming for me in the form of an Easter Day breakfast and celebration. As we all got ready to dig in, my dad handed out sparkling juice to the kids and champagne to the adults, and made a toast: "Here's to Steve, his new heart and the wonderful healing grace of our Lord!"

Then Sara toasted, "Here's to Cindy, a model of love, strength and courage."

It was a special day all around.

While playing catch-up at work and trying to manage all that was coming my way, there were two additional personal events on my calendar that I had vowed not to miss, regardless of what was happening. One was for a surprise deep sea fishing trip to Destin, Florida for my dad on his 80th birthday. The other was a Memorial Day foot race, the Cotton Row Run, which my dad, my younger brother, Mark, and I were planning to run along with other family members and friends. I had been looking forward to both events, and I wasn't about to use my heart transplant as an excuse to bow out.

Sara had managed to keep Dad in the dark about the fishing trip, so when we told him about it, he was flabbergasted and delighted. It turned out to be a blast. Besides my dad and me, the "crew" included Mark and his two sons, Will and Wesley; his father-in-law, Dr. Tytula, a retired professor; and Cindy's brother-in-law, Stephen, and his son, Bryan. The weather was perfect, sunny and not too hot, and the Gulf seas were smooth as glass. When Captain Ken of the "Just-B-Cause" heard it was my dad's 80th birthday, he put out into deeper water, adding an extra two hours to the ride. We caught our limit of amberjack within a half hour before we had to head back to port.

Then it was time to put my new heart to the test in the Cotton Row Run. I had been walking two miles per day three times a week, but following the doctors' discharge orders from UAB, hadn't been able to jog or run until just a few weeks before the 5K race (a little more than three miles). I really wasn't sure if I would be able to make it all the way on the hilly terrain of the route in the springtime heat.

On race day, our team assembled on the street near the starting gate in downtown Huntsville. After some instructions from the officials, chatting and last minute stretching, the gun fired and we were off. On the initial stretch of five-lane road lined by tall buildings—tall by Huntsville's standards, that is—I started to pull ahead of Mark and Dad a bit. Glancing over my shoulder, I was pretty certain that the two of them were going to stick together for the entire race, and decided to go ahead alone. As I took a left turn onto Lincoln Street, the rest of the field and I were blasted by the full mid-morning sun and I was feeling the heat. Sweat started to stream down my body.

As I passed the one-mile marker, a race volunteer shouted out the elapsed time, "Thirteen minutes, eight seconds."

"I'm on pace," I thought, but wondered how I was going to manage to make it to the end. It felt like I had run half the race with more than two thirds to go. This was much tougher than running on a treadmill inside the air-conditioned Spain Rehabilitation Center.

After turning right onto Meridian Drive, still in full sunlight, I saw respite ahead: big tall shade trees lining both sides of Walker Avenue, a neighborhood of beautiful antique homes. Passing under the trees was a welcome treat, as were the cooling showers provided by a couple of residents who were standing on the sidewalk with garden hoses and fanning water in a high arc onto the street.

As I turned right onto White Street, I overtook two women. One was quite athletic and running backward, shouting encouragement like a drill sergeant to the other, who was slightly overweight and struggling. "This is your goal, this is what you wanted to achieve today! So, come on! Don't walk, try running again!" she urged her friend on.

I turned around, too, peddled backward for several steps and said, "Hey, I just had a heart transplant three and a half months ago. If I can do it, you can, too!"

"Are you kidding?" they both said in unison.

"Nope. Keep pushing yourself!"

As I turned around and made my way up the street, I could hear the trainee shouting after me, "I'm running now, I'm running!"

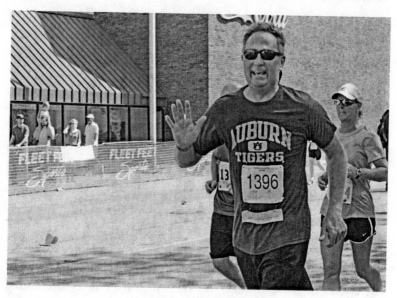

Cotton Row Run 2012

At the second mile marker, another volunteer called out, "Twenty-six minutes, forty seconds."

Two thirds of the way, and I was not too far off pace. But I was having second thoughts. The heat was really bearing down on me, and I began to wonder if I had charged out of the gate too early after my heart transplant. While I didn't have any of the cardiac symptoms I had suffered in the past, I was exhausted, hot, and I could feel my heart beating rapidly in my chest. Several times, I was forced to drop my pace to a brisk walk for 30 seconds or more to let my heart rate settle down a bit. That helped enough for me to continue through downtown Huntsville. So did a few more showers from hoses on the sidelines and water handed to me in cone-shaped paper cups.

On the final stretch of the race, the tall buildings provided some shade, and surprisingly, a few cool, refreshing gusts of wind swept across the street. Still, I was about to slow to another fast walk, when I heard my good friend Tanner yelling from the sidewalk, "Go Steve, you can do it! You are almost to the finish line!"

Tanner himself was still recovering from a terrible bicycle accident that had left him almost paralyzed from the neck down several years earlier. His recovery took longer, but was no less miraculous than mine, and he now walks with a limp and has some limited motion in his hands. With his encouragement, I knew I wasn't going to stop until I hit the finish line.

And I made it, with enough energy to continue down Clinton Avenue and past the parking lot where we had gathered less than an hour earlier, slowing my pace to a walk. I appreciated the cheers of more friends and family. Mark and Dad finished a few minutes behind me, holding hands and waving in unison at the crowd. It wasn't long before we were all assembled and chatting about the race, which I completed in 40 minutes and four seconds, 14 seconds better than the target I had set for myself. For an engineer like me, to whom figures really matter, it represented a significant margin of victory. The photo of me crossing the finish line made the ten o'clock news as part of a poignant story about the man with a heart transplant who conquered the Cotton Row 5K.

But life with a new heart was not just a one-sided success story. It took me more than two months to become comfortable with and accept my condition.

In the fall, I had a week-long bout with bronchitis. Although it passed without mishap, I felt quite emotional. In fact, I got more worried and scared than I did during the time of my heart failure and transplant operation. It was as if all the fears I had bottled up inside came pouring out at once.

The experience certainly made me pay more attention to taking care of myself, especially when going out. At church, when greeting others, I'd hug and shake hands, but then use a pocket-sized bottle of sanitizer. I tried to be the first in line for Communion, knowing that the pastor took a piece of bread, dipped it into the cup and then touched everyone's palm. I didn't touch the offering plate when it came around but let people to either side of me handle it. Since I was in charge of church finances, I'd handle the plate after the service, but sanitize my hands quickly afterward.

At gas station pumps, I'd get a paper towel to hold the dispensing handle, press buttons with my pinky and then wash or sanitize my hands.

I appreciate the Handi Wipes dispenser Publix provides at its grocery stores and would get two—one for each hand—to drape over the shopping cart handle.

In restaurants, I learned to identify and avoid "where the germs are"—door handles, waiting list pagers, menus, breadbaskets, lemons squeezed into drinks, unwrapped silverware, salt and pepper shakers, and other condiment containers. Just about everyone grabs the underside of the chair when scooting closer to the table, so I don't do that anymore.

So when we went to Rosie's, our favorite Mexican restaurant, for example, once we had been seated, I'd go wash my hands before enjoying the chips and salsa. Sometimes, I'd get my hands clean and run into a friend on the way back to the table who wanted to shake hands, requiring a return trip to the bathroom. One day, it happened twice at a Five Guys burger joint!

Public restrooms presented a special challenge, especially the older, manual ones. There'd be flush handles, faucet handles, soap dispensers, and air dryer buttons. After washing my hands, it was easy to forget and grab the handle to shut off the water, potentially recontaminating my hands. Not to mention touching the air dryer button and the door handle on the way out. That's when my little bottle of sanitizer came in very handy.

Fortunately, I was busy on all fronts, and the summer and early fall flew by. With work demands, frequent visits to the Kirklin Clinic for checkups, Anna participating in a summer program at Baylor University in Houston, Brooke moving to Yuma, Arizona, to start her first job, and assisting Lindsey and Jay in setting up their first home in Katy, a suburb of Houston, there was never a dull moment. I certainly had no time to feel disenfranchised from the events of the past three and a half years. Life was coming at me at a rapid-fire pace, and I liked it that way.

Late in the fall, two scheduled events forced me to step back, however, and take the time to look at my journey from a bigger vantage point. Gary Bond, organizer of Asbury's Men's Power Lunch, a periodic gathering of about 50 men, asked me to speak to the group in November; and Brother Marcus asked me to speak to his Sunday school class in December.

To get ready, I had to reflect on my story from tachycardia to transplant, and everything came into sharper focus. I prepared handouts, talking points and notes. Both groups had asked me to speak for 15 to 30 minutes, but the first dry run of my talk in the basement, with Cindy standing in for the audience, was almost 50 minutes long! I was still so close to the experience that I wanted to crowd everything that had happened to me into the presentation. How do I tell my story giving just enough information to keep the audience engaged without shortchanging His message? I wanted to be sure listeners walked away energized and convinced as much in the power of prayer as I am today. Cindy critiquing my practice sessions helped greatly, and I eventually delivered both talks successfully, and within the allotted time.

During the presentations I encountered a new challenge due to my new heart. I started off sounding much more nervous and shaky than I felt. Doing some research on my own, I learned that a transplanted heart was denervated—no longer connected to the brain—and beats faster than normal. It was controlled more by adrenaline and other chemicals in the bloodstream than my natural brain functions. Running as high as 140 beats per minute when I began speaking, it made me come off sounding on edge, which made the audience uneasy. So I bought a finger tip pulse oximeter at a drugstore. It measures heart rate and I use it as an icebreaker. Calling on volunteers in the audience, I compare my heart rate to theirs and start my speech with, "So, imagine if you were up here running on a treadmill until your heart rate got as high as mine, and then I asked you to deliver a speech!" From that point on, everyone seems at ease with the sound of my new, shaky voice and can enjoy the rest of my talk.

On the Sunday prior to Christmas break, before the morning service got underway at Asbury, Brother Marcus told me he had something to give me. Afterward, I became engrossed in my routine to gather and secure the offering from the pulpit, and we didn't cross paths. Because I vacationed with my family over Christmas in St. Augustine again this year, it wasn't until two Sundays later that Marcus and I caught up with one another.

After he finished greeting members leaving the sanctuary, we headed to his compact truck in the parking lot. From the front seat, he produced a gift bag with my name on the outside and handed it to me, beaming. It was heavy. When I finally managed to sift through the wrapping paper, I found a bronze-colored sculpture, a beautiful set of praying hands. The message inscribed at the bottom read, "MFL 1980," his initials and the year he had cast the sculpture. I immediately got emotional holding this extraordinary keepsake, which he had made with his own hands years before he founded Asbury Church, the year I met Cindy!

Walking back to the church, he told me that the gift was his response to my sharing my story at the Power Lunch and again one evening at the home of Asbury founding members, Herschel and Marge Jordan, who were hosting about 25 couples at their annual Sunday school party.

We hugged, and I felt deeply humbled to receive this gift from our founding pastor, the one who had the original vision of a new church in Madison, who led a flock of parishioners to raise funds and construct the first building on Hughes Road, who reeled me and Cindy into his church, and who instilled the importance of prayer within me.

The praying hands now sit on the corner of my desk, glimmering under the lamp, clearly visible from my prayer chair.

POSTLUDE

PRAYER AND GRACE

When I reflect on my journey up to now, my thoughts often turn to the suffering our Lord, Jesus Christ, took upon Himself. In order to know His Father's will, and eventually accept it, even He had to pray often, sometimes all night and with heartfelt energy. If He had to invest so much time in prayer, how can we know His agenda for us without praying—either at all or as a priority in our daily lives?

During the events described in these pages, I did not go to heaven and back, nor did I see heaven and know firsthand that it is real. What I did experience was His presence, intimate and personal, in my home and workplace, along the beach, in medical facilities and other places where He decided to appear to me at times and in response to my prayers, at times without being called. In the process I have changed from that scrappy youngster and young man who had little interest in getting to know Him, to a mature, faith-filled man. I've learned that anyone can tap into His abundant grace by engaging in the power of prayer. I am happy to tell my story to others—the parable of a man who asked God for help during the most difficult of times and received His grace. I'm now completely comfortable and thankful for the gift of a new heart because I now, in a very personal way, know that He is real and works through others and on His own. Yes, He listens and responds, although His answers may not be the ones we've been expecting or hoping for. And so His purpose may not initially be evident, may not seem like a comfortable fit, but I have come to realize that it has been custom tailored for me. I have found that experiencing God's purpose through His answers to my prayers, which lie outside the confines of my understanding, is grace indeed.

For more information
and to contact Steve Burcham go to

www.prayerandgracethebook.com

CPSIA information can be obtained at www.ICGtesting.com
Printed in the USA
LVOW120720110313

323504LV00003B/5/P